The Elimination Diet

Workbook

A Personal Approach to Determining Your Food Allergies

MAGGIE MOON, MS, RD

ULYSSES PRESS

Published in the U.S. by:
Ulysses Press
P.O. Box 3440
Berkeley, CA 94703
www.ulyssespress.com

ISBN13: 978-1-61243-300-4
Library of Congress Control Number: 2013957325

Acquisitions editor: Katherine Furman
Managing editor: Claire Chun
Editor: Kathy Kaiser
Proofreader: Lauren Harrison
Index: Sayre Van Young
Front cover design: Double R Design
Cover art: wine © lenetstan/shutterstock.com; walnuts © Donatella Tandelli/shutterstock.com; fish © Sergiy Zavgorodny/shutterstock.com; strawberries © DenisNata/shutterstock.com; eggs © apiguide/shutterstock.com; lobster © Edward Westmacott/shutterstock.com; bread © v.s.anandhakrishna/shutterstock.com; sesame seeds © Olaf Speier/shutterstock.com; Swiss cheese © Africa Studio/shutterstock.com; apples © PhotoSGH/shutterstock.com; corn © diane diederich/istock.com; steak © Jacek Chabraszewski/shutterstock.com; soybeans © Suzifoo/istock.com; watermelon © Markus Mainka/shutterstock.com; peanuts © Markus Mainka/shutterstock.com; tomatoes © Robyn Mackenzie/shutterstock.com; kiwi © LI CHAOSHU/shutterstock.com; salami © al1962/shutterstock.com; pistachios © Christian Jung/shutterstock.com; cherries © Alberto Zornetta/shutterstock.com; oysters © V. J. Matthew/shutterstock.com; spinach © Dionisvera/shutterstock.com; figs © kaband/shutterstock.com; blue cheese © AlexussK/shutterstock.com; wheat © illustrart/shutterstock.com
Interior design: Jake Flaherty
Illustration page 21 © La Gorda/shutterstock.com

10 9 8 7 6 5 4 3 2

For my mom and dad, Dr. and Mrs. Moon,
who nourished me and taught me how food can heal. For my siblings, Ahrie, Gurie, Suerie,
and Kahmyong, one of whom lives with a peanut allergy, and all of whom lived with me
and my food intolerance. Finally, for my husband Fred, one of the best eaters I know.

Contents

Author's Note

The major nutrition problems of our day can be solved with basic shifts in eating habits. Implementing these simple changes can be complex, but the guidance is simple: more vegetables, more fruit, more whole grains, a handful of nuts a day, seafood twice a week, lean proteins, and don't go crazy with booze or butter. But this is advice for the luckier ones, who have no more to deal with than, say, navigating the modern food system, which seems tailor-made to keep us overweight.

Imagine that in addition to the basic challenge of eating healthfully in the Western world, you had a particularly adversarial relationship with food. What if food—which is supposed to nurture your physical well-being, cement your cultural and social bonds, provide pleasure, and so much more—actually caused you distress and discomfort? What if it were the root of, or at least a contributing factor to, your fatigue, hives, rashes, stomachaches, migraine headaches, asthma, coughs, bloating, gas, or diarrhea? And what if you weren't sure which foods were triggering your symptoms?

Although the percentage of people with food allergies (when the body's immune system has an inappropriate reaction to a food) or food intolerances (most often a negative digestive reaction to a food) is dwarfed by the percentage of those without them, the number of human beings suffering from food sensitivities (encompassing both food allergies and food intolerances) is significant. In the United States, an estimated 5 percent of the population has food allergies (about 15 million), and 16 percent of Americans (nearly 60 million) self-report food intolerances (though blind tests suggest its closer to 1 to 2 percent). Because the relationship between foods and symptoms is incompletely understood and varies a great deal according to the individual, diagnosis can difficult. In conjunction with a thorough medical history, the gold standard for diagnosis is the subject of this book: the elimination diet.

If possible, I highly recommend that you work with a credible and supportive health care team to deal with your food sensitivities. They can provide the face-to-face guidance and individualized support you may need. Many registered dietitians have expertise in this area. But if for whatever reason you do not do this, I hope this book will help guide you through at-home versions of the elimination diet that can be done safely with minimal risk to the nutritional adequacy of your diet, and that can potentially have profound benefits for your quality of life.

My graduate training in nutrition on my way to becoming a registered dietitian means that I approach the topic of elimination diets with academic rigor and professional responsibility. I am also empathetic and want to help. I've lived with a food intolerance for most of my life Although my lactose intolerance is now very manageable, I know how disruptive a food intolerance can be.

In addition, my graduate program at Columbia University demanded that we put concepts into practice. We tasted every liquid nutritional supplement we might ever have to prescribe in a hospital setting (not a five-star dining experience). We spent time on just about every basic therapeutic diet, popular diet, and even a food stamp diet—all to "get a taste" of what our patients were going through. We juggled classes, work, family, and diets that were restrictive in one way or another. This means that the tips and tools that I've created are practical, rooted in reality, and helpful.

The darker side of popularizing any specialized diet that cuts out foods is that it could promote disordered eating. It is in no way my intention or desire to do this. Quite the opposite. I come at this with a love of food and want to help you restore your diet to something you enjoy and that supports your vitality and good health.

Food is not just fuel. It is also delicious, it is fun, it can call forth creativity in its preparation, it represents caring, and it is healing. Thank goodness we are omnivores! We have many choices when it comes to nourishing the body. Let's discover the foods that disagree with you, put them aside, and discover a world of flavors that you can safely enjoy.

Wishing you good health,
Maggie Moon, MS, RD

Introduction

The elimination diet is about helping you feel better by identifying what foods are causing your symptoms. It's a way back to enjoying food and getting the nourishment you need and deserve to support a healthful lifestyle. The elimination diet is gaining in popularity, though it has been known to the dietetics and medical communities for a long time as a way to figure out what food ails you. There is a lot of information out there, often conflicting or incomplete, on how you should go about this diet. This book is a guide to conducting an elimination diet that can be done safely at home, with minimal risk of depriving you of important nutrients in the long term.

Who This Book Is For and Who It Is Not For

This book is for you if you have a hunch that something in your diet is preventing you from feeling your best. It's also for you if you are interested in resetting your palate and sharpening your senses to sugar, salt, and processed foods through a few weeks of simple eating.

It's not for you if you know you have a food allergy that causes anaphylaxis, in which case you should be working closely with your health care team, including a qualified dietitian, to manage your condition.

This book was written with US adults in mind; it is not intended for use with infants or children. Food allergies and intolerances are not uncommon in these age groups, but infants and children should be treated under a physician's supervision.

Finally, this book is not for you if you are pregnant or breast-feeding. You should be following the guidance of your physician and health care team.

What This Book Is and Is Not

This book provides background information on select food allergies and food intolerances, and it guides you through a couple of basic versions of elimination diets. If intolerances are highly suspected or uncovered, this book cannot provide you with full, ongoing support; it does not include a lifelong diet for your individual needs. There are many well-qualified allergists and registered dietitians with expertise in food sensitivities. The resources section provides information to point you in the right direction.

The Book in Detail

PART ONE starts with an overview of misconceptions about elimination diets and then describes the origins of elimination diets, how they work, and where they can fill in the gaps left by modern testing. This part also provides a brief overview of how the gut works (it's truly a magical place!).

PART TWO dives into what is going on when the body reacts poorly to a food. It describes the most common foods that trigger symptoms caused by allergies, intolerances, inflammation, digestive disorders, and more. This discussion answers the question of why you would want to embark on an elimination diet (to feel better!). Because the elimination diet can be challenging, it is helpful to know what is going on in your body and why you are making changes to your diet. The more you know about why you're doing something, the better able you are to stick to it.

PART THREE is a crash course in elimination diets. It describes two types of elimination diets and provides all the information you'll need to follow an elimination diet, including doing a baseline assessment, planning meals, avoiding certain foods, reintroducing them into your diet, and evaluating your body's reactions to them.

PART FOUR is designed to make the elimination diet as easy as possible for you. It has everything I want to equip you with, given that I won't be able to see you personally for nutritional counseling. Its tips and tools include meal plans, grocery lists, and recipes, which will be especially useful when you're just starting out and have eliminated so many foods. This part also includes tools, such as kitchen checklists, food and symptom tracker worksheets, tips on how to identify hidden ingredients on a food label, reference sheets for the foods you need to avoid during the elimination phase of the diet, worksheets to guide you through the challenge phase, meal planning guidelines for the maintenance phase, and more.

In the resources section, you'll find my recommendations for further study and action, whether you want to seek additional information, find a qualified health care professional, or join a supportive community that understands food allergies and intolerances.

This book aims to be a credible yet approachable guide to the elimination diet that will help you clarify the relationship between food and its effects on *your* body. You will be in tune with how your food choices influence how you feel. The elimination diet is not a one-size-fits-all diet; it is a diet that you personalize. While so many people eat mindlessly, you will be empowered to help heal yourself. With the elimination diet, you apply the scientific method to discover what works and what doesn't when it comes to the most magnificent machine you'll ever get to operate: your body.

PART ONE
Why Try an Elimination Diet?

CHAPTER 1

Pop Culture, the True Origins of the Elimination Diet, and How It Works

Pop Culture and Where It Goes Wrong

The elimination diet has recently made headlines via starlets and self-proclaimed health gurus, making it seem like the latest fad diet. It is definitely the answer to all your problems—at least for today's news cycle. It's also been called a cleanse diet or detox diet.

Have you heard the expression, They know just enough to be dangerous? Although there might be some truth in the advice to avoid certain foods, that advice means nothing without putting it in the context of your total diet, your body, your life, and your health. When a celeb tells you not to eat, say, grapefruit, does that mean grapefruit is bad for everyone? Unless *your* body doesn't like it, why deprive yourself of a perfectly good source of vitamin C, fiber, and antioxidants? People like and need options in their diets.

Here's another example. A certain celebrity eliminated gluten from her diet and lost a lot of weight. Does that mean gluten causes weight gain? Or that avoiding it is the secret to weight loss? Don't be fooled. Eliminating any food from the diet might have that effect at first, especially if it's a big part of the regular diet. It's also true that a lot of food contains gluten, including junk food. If cutting out gluten means cutting out junk, then it's a healthy choice. But today, there are plenty of gluten-free junk foods, too, which further complicates the story. Only by putting food choices in the context of your total diet and your individual health can you determine what works for you.

Choosing to avoid a food makes it that much more difficult to eat a varied, balanced, and healthy diet. Not impossible, of course, but it does make the job more complicated. Cutting out foods for the sake of today's fad may also be a sign of disordered eating. Don't be taken in by gimmicks. We are omnivores and are meant to eat a variety of foods to sustain us and keep us healthy. When our bodies don't agree with all the foods we put into them, that—not pop culture figures—is something we should listen to.

If you choose to follow an elimination diet, do it for you, do it for health. Do it to feel good and be in tune with your body. The elimination diet, when undertaken for the right reasons, can transform your relationship with food, helping you eat in a way that will make you feel good and revitalized.

Origins

Elimination diets probably date back untold centuries. If you got sick after eating something, the thinking likely went, you'd feel better if you avoided it. However, the elimination diet as a formal therapy for food sensitivities has its roots in 1920s medicine. Since then, many variations on the theme have been proposed to solve a variety of ailments that don't respond to standard treatment.

Food is the single biggest wild card in how your body interacts with the world. When you eat a food, you invite the outside world to interact with your body in an intimate way. Food breaks down into chemicals that contribute to or detract from optimal function, and can affect how you breathe, think, move, stay healthy, and thrive. It might also contribute to inflammation, allergies, intolerances, and chronic disease. Considering how much "data" the digestive system (aka the gut) has to work through, it's no wonder that the main system involved in how the body interacts with food is one of the largest and most complex, complete with its own immune system.

A food sensitivity could potentially result in:

- Abdominal pain
- Anxiety
- Asthma
- Bloating
- Chronic congestion
- Constipation
- Coughing
- Depression
- Diarrhea

- Difficulty breathing
- Earache
- Eczema
- Gas
- Headaches from fatigue or migraines
- Hives
- Insomnia
- Irritable bowel syndrome

- Itchiness
- Joint or muscle pain
- Nausea
- Rash
- Runny nose
- Stomach cramping
- Swelling
- Vomiting
- Wheezing, or, in severe cases, anaphylaxis

One food could trigger any one or more of these symptoms, which means the standard medical model doesn't work here: one-test-one-disease, diagnose, treat, feel better. And that's where the rationale for an elimination diet comes in: Identify and eliminate the cause, and you eliminate the symptoms. Because there was no simple, reliable test to identify which of the many foods a person ate could be causing the symptoms, the elimination diet emerged as a way to do just that.

How It Works

As a diagnostic tool, an elimination diet can help identify foods that are causing negative symptoms, such as those mentioned in the preceding section. In contrast, elimination diets as therapy are used to eliminate symptom-triggering foods that need to be avoided for life. This book focuses on the elimination diet as a diagnostic tool that helps you discover what foods are causing your symptoms. (Part Three of this book is devoted to the ins and outs of elimination diets, but this is the essence of what they do.)

For food allergies, the *Guidelines for the Diagnosis and Management of Food Allergy in the United States: Summary of the NIAID-Sponsored Expert Panel Report* from the National Institute of Allergy and Infectious Diseases says that elimination diets can identify foods causing an allergy and can confirm a food allergy. The *Guidelines* recommends elimination diets as one of the main diagnostic tools for specific disorders that are associated with food allergies. These are food-protein-induced enterocolitis syndrome (FPIES), food-protein-induced allergic protocolitis, allergic contact dermatitis, systemic contact dermatitis, and eosinophilic esophagitis (EoE). The first two conditions are infant disorders and won't be discussed in this book. Contact dermatitis (e.g., to nickel) and EoE can occur in adults, and an elimination diet can help identify the trigger foods (see chapters on nickel sensitivity, and EoE, both in part 2).

Elimination diets may also be helpful for the wide range of food sensitivities that are hard to detect by lab tests for one reason or another (e.g., test results are hard to read or no tests exist that uniquely identify a particular food sensitivity).

Benefits of an Elimination Diet

If done correctly, and food is indeed related to your complaints, an elimination diet can identify your symptom-triggering foods. Once identified and eliminated, you will experience a lot of relief. Improved symptoms is probably the number one benefit. It's about feeling better and living a life in good health.

There may also be some fringe benefits: weight loss, palate resetting, or healthy habits. The elimination diet is not meant to be used a weight loss diet, but weight loss is common when you take more control over your diet and become vigilant about what you let into your body. The goal is health, not weight loss, but you may find that they go hand in hand. Also, because the elimination diet is very different from the usual American diet, chances are that your palate will change. It will be reset to be sensitive to and prefer natural flavors and textures. You may find that you don't prefer as much salt or sugar in your foods, or that you no longer want fried foods or junk foods. Finally, the time and care you take with your food may be a shift from your regular habits. Finding time to make your own healthy food, within the context of your busy life, is a skill you can take with you that is a benefit beyond anything the elimination diet can offer on its own.

Interview with Penny B.

Penny, the first elimination diet you went on was when you were in elementary school. You did another just this year at age thirty-four, due to the reemergence of your symptoms. Looking back, what stands out in your memory in terms of what was hardest to cope with?

Some of the hardships I remember are the chronic discomfort, feeling left out at school or at birthday parties and disliking the foods I was allowed to eat (rice cakes, carob soy milk—I still wrinkle my nose at these foods!). Before the diet, I loved toast with butter, grilled cheese, chocolate, etc. (I still love these foods.) But the truth is that I would have done anything to improve my physical condition.

Did the elimination diet work? Did you figure out your trigger foods?

The diet eventually cleared up my skin enough to take an extensive allergy test, which showed a violent allergy to eggs and moderate allergies to dairy and wheat. I avoided dairy and wheat for another two years, and eggs for another fifteen years (until I was in my early twenties). The doctors thought that eating eggs too early in my childhood had thrown my entire immune system out of whack, creating temporary secondary allergies to wheat and dairy.

What's your diet like now?

I have some clear allergies to foods (dairy, shellfish, etc.) that I avoid, and in an effort to keep inflammation to a minimum, I avoid pretty much anything that I've had a reaction to on any allergy test or that seems to correlate with any kind of allergic response. I also have a contact dermatitis allergy to nickel, and a few years ago I went on an experimental low-nickel diet, which seemed to improve conditions somewhat. That diet was very inconvenient, so now I just try to avoid the foods that are highest in nickel.

What would you tell someone about to embark on an elimination diet about what to expect?

I've done severely restricted diets only out of desperation because I was so physically uncomfortable, so I easily would say they were worth it, even if all they did was suggest the lack of some additional food allergy (as was the case with the lamb and rice diet). Better to know than not know! I do think that for people with chronic pain or discomfort, a restricted diet can sometimes create an illusion of control to compensate for the lack of control over one's general health. It makes me wonder if in extreme cases, this tendency might start to approach an eating disorder. I try to be self-aware in this regard.

Thank you so much for sharing your experiences and your insights. You are right that diet manipulation, when done for the wrong reasons, could potentially lead to disordered eating, and that is a real concern. I think you're right that an elimination diet is truly worth it when it helps people feel better.

Penny B. (name has been changed for privacy), is a thirty-four-year-old woman from California.

Challenges of an Elimination Diet

For most, the possibility of symptom relief is motivation enough, no matter how hard the diet. But it is challenging to make many changes to the diet at the same time and to be vigilant about tracking what you eat and how you feel for several weeks. Further, the changes to the diet are restrictions, and it can be hard to stick to a diet that limits your options.

CLINICAL INSIGHTS

Expert Interview with Robin Foroutan, MS, RDN

What is your area of specialty?

Integrative- and functional-medicine-based nutrition therapy, specializing in digestive health; diet support for infectious, neurological, and toxicity-related disease protocols; and a general "food as medicine" approach to health and healing.

What is your experience with using elimination diets? People seem to have many different versions. What kinds of elimination diets have you worked with?

I personalize all my protocols depending on various factors, such as symptoms and overall health status, ability and willingness to change, but I typically start by pulling some of the usual suspects: wheat, gluten, corn, soy. And I'll usually do a dairy challenge (remove dairy for a few weeks and methodically reintroduce to assess tolerance to casein, whey, etc.). I might also recommend avoiding other common allergens, like peanuts, shellfish, eggs, chicken, and beef, especially if the diet is very monotonous with any one food.

For those experiencing extreme, persistent bloating, I may use a FODMAPS-based elimination diet. I also use diet protocols similar to the GAPS diet, or the Specific Carbohydrate Diet, which eliminates all grains, soy, sugar, and high-lactose dairy foods. The intention is always to reintroduce the eliminated foods in order to detect which foods a person is truly sensitive to. Typically, people may be reactive to many foods initially, but tolerance can improve after a period of avoidance and a nutritional protocol to support gut healing. In cases where there are multiple sensitivities and the person reports that they're becoming more sensitive to an increasing number of foods, that is indicative of an underlying issue.

The bottom line is food sensitivities are generally a function of a compromised digestive system.

How are the mediator release test (MRT), an experimental test for food sensitivities, and the accompanying lifestyle eating and performance (LEAP) program regarded by allergists and registered dietitians who work in the area of food allergies and intolerances?

I can't speak for all allergists, but I personally haven't crossed paths with any allergists who use LEAP/ MRT testing, and many practitioners are understandably skeptical, since the existing published

If you don't already cook at home regularly—and even if you do—you'll be taking time to learn how to prepare foods that may be different from what you know. And if you need to work on your kitchen skills, this can be an extra challenge. Relatedly, it may be hard to eat out at restaurants, while traveling, or socially at friends' homes because chances are that you will not be able to find the foods you need to eat.

All these changes can also have an effect on anyone you live with. Your spouse, kids, friends, and roommates will be affected, especially if you're the one who buys or prepares food for them.

data is far from conclusive. However, it's important to keep practice-based evidence in mind as well. I have shared patients with allergists who have used antigen leukocyte antibody test (ALCAT) panels, and who may run Immunoglobulin G-based (IgG, a type of antibody) food sensitivity testing. I believe IgG has its limitations, because results are dependent upon the integrity of the intestinal mucosa, and most people we see have some degree of increased intestinal permeability. On the whole, allergists focus on Immunoglobulin E-based (IgE, a type of antibody) reactions, which are considered true allergies. It is obviously important to detect potentially life-threatening allergic reactions to foods, and elimination diets based on IgE improve symptoms in many people. However, there are so many different immune- and nonimmune-mediated reactions to food, and no one test captures them all, which is why so many other testing methods exist and why elimination diets are so useful. I find that elimination diets are the gold standard when assessing non-IgE food sensitivities.

I'm not a certified LEAP therapist (CLT) or registered dietitian (RD), but I do think the test has its place, and I may run the panel to identify possible reactive foods that may be triggering inflammation. With that said, I've also had patients follow elimination diets based on MRT results with mild benefits or no noticeable benefits at all. So I think the test can be used as a good tool, but it doesn't exclusively guide all of my elimination protocols.

If a good friend—who has no food allergies that she knows of—were adamant about trying something on her own at home before going to a clinician, and she wanted to experiment with her diet for a couple of weeks on her own to see if she could figure out if food was leading to her symptoms, what advice would you give her?

Most people have some degree of food sensitivity, and most people are not aware of it. It would really depend on the specific kinds of symptoms she experiences: digestive discomfort, muscle or joint pain, fatigue (especially fatigue after meals). I'd first see if there were junk ingredients still in her diet—food colorings, artificial sweeteners, MSG, artificial flavorings and preservatives, etc. Even just clearing the nonfood edibles from the diet can yield great results. Beyond that, I'd probably recommend trying gluten-free/dairy-free, but without incorporating processed gluten-free foods, since those products introduce lots of starches and flours that are likely not already in the diet and can derail an elimination diet. I'd also look at the foods she's eating most frequently, since that can provide clues to food sensitivities. Beyond that, I'd recommend that she work with someone to help guide her, because there's only so much a person can handle on his or her own. It's also helpful and comforting to partner with someone trustworthy and experienced in guiding people through elimination diets.

Robin Foroutan, MS, RDN, is an integrative medicine dietitian-nutritionist.

The elimination diet phase takes two weeks or as long as it takes for symptoms to subside. However, during the week prior to it, you are gathering baseline data. And the challenge phase can be several weeks more, depending on how many challenge foods you have to test. On the upside, by the end of the two-

---

CLINICAL INSIGHTS

Expert Interview with Scott H. Sicherer, MD

As a clinician, are there things that you see again and again that patients struggle with when it comes to the elimination diet?

When diagnostic elimination is being undertaken, we have to take into consideration the natural ups and downs of symptoms and other factors that may influence symptom patterns, aside from the diet. For example, if a new medication is used at the same time that the diet is changed, we may not know which intervention improved the symptoms.

Elimination diets for food allergy require education about the avoidance of certain foods, meaning label reading, understanding cross-contact issues in food preparation, and so on. Otherwise, mistakes could misinform the results. There also is a difference in treatment versus diagnostic elimination because diagnostic elimination is short term. Long-term elimination has to consider the impact on nutrition.

Many people are probably trying long-term elimination diets on their own without medical supervision. What do you think of this consumer trend?

Food allergy impacts quality of life. Elimination diets carry social, emotional, and nutritional risks, among others. If we are discussing true food allergies, it is important to get a diagnosis, because a food allergy can be life-threatening. You want to be avoiding the right trigger foods and not avoiding innocent ones, and you want to be prepared to treat any severe allergic reactions.

There is also some evidence that long-term unnecessary elimination of allergens could result in increasing the risk of developing a true allergy to the avoided food. While this is relatively unusual, it is another reason to work with a doctor when dealing with food allergies.

By trying a long-term elimination diet without a doctor, what might people be missing out on?

It is crucial to talk to a doctor. Maybe the symptoms are being misinterpreted as related to food, when in fact the symptoms are caused by some serious underlying illness. Experimenting with dietary changes without a discussion with your doctor may delay a diagnosis, and result in losing valuable time for treatment.

There seem to be a lot of different ideas about what should and shouldn't be included in an elimination diet. Ideally, an elimination diet would be individually designed for someone.

There are no set diets to try for an allergy elimination diet, though it could be a diet that is devoid of most common allergens. Still, there is no set elimination diet as a one size fits all.

Scott H. Sicherer, MD, is professor of pediatrics and a researcher at the Jaffe Food Allergy Institute at Mount Sinai in New York and author of Food Allergies: A Complete Guide to Eating When Your Life Depends on It *(Baltimore: Johns Hopkins University Press, 2013).*

week elimination diet, you will know what you're doing. The diet might be a little mundane, but it will no longer be the challenge that it was at the beginning.

The good news is that being ready for these challenges and having strategies to deal with them can help make them easier. Maybe not easy, but easier. And that's what part 4 of this book is all about: tips and tools to help you manage the process before, during, and after the elimination diet.

Professional Support for an Elimination Diet

As with most things in life, the shortcut to success is to work with a teacher or coach who shows you the way. For an elimination diet, you would want to seek out and work directly with a qualified registered dietitian. It really helps to have that personalized support from someone who has helped many others on a similar journey. If that's not available to you, a book, such as this one, can be helpful.

If you know that food causes anaphylaxis for you or you have already been diagnosed with a food allergy, you should be working with a qualified team of health care professionals, including an allergist and a registered dietitian. It is crucial to talk to your physician and perhaps an allergist initially to rule out conditions that are caused by something other than food.

Further, if you have a history of anaphylactic shock, disordered eating (e.g., anorexia or bulimia), a self-guided elimination diet is not for you. Lastly, if you are on any medications that are diet-sensitive (e.g., Coumadin dosages are set based on your regular vitamin K intake), you'll want to work with your physician before making any changes to your diet.

CHAPTER 2

How the Gut Works

The gut is the intersection of food and the body. To understand all the ways in which food, provider of nourishment and so many pleasures, might instead cause discomfort, displeasure, and even disease, let's start with the basics. Food is a foreign substance. It is the primary way the outside world gets in. It is certainly one of the most intimate ways we interact with our world; and, unlike the air we breathe, we have a diversity of choices regarding what to put in our mouths. Following is a brief overview of the digestive system, end to end, and how the body interacts with food along the way. This will provide you with the foundational background to understand what is going on in your gut.

The digestive system—unlike the Internet—actually is a series of tubes, also called the digestive tract. Other names for the whole system are the gastrointestinal tract (GI tract, or just GI, for short), the gut, and the bowel. The tubes of the digestive system are everywhere your lunchtime sandwich goes: They start at the mouth, go down the esophagus, into the stomach, into the small and large intestines, with a final stop at the rectum before exiting out the anus. All along these tubes is a lining of muscles that help mechanically break food down and move it along, as if the food were on an assembly line. Last but not least, the pancreas and the liver (plus the liver's sidekick, the gallbladder) provide important digestive aids that get piped into the intestines when needed.

Essentially, the digestive system extracts nutrients large and small from food (by the way, when I say "food," I'm including beverages, too—basically anything that goes down the hatch). The gut transforms the food you put into your mouth into its smallest pieces, so that these bits can fit into the bloodstream, which then carries the bits to the rest of the body to build, nourish, and energize the body for everything from running a mile to writing an essay. This probably sounds familiar; it's the digestive system as it is described in the classroom.

But that's not all. The second major job the digestive system has is coping with the barrage of foreign substances to which it is exposed. In other words, it serves as your bodyguard by providing a physical and immunity barrier to microorganisms, any nonfood things you have accidentally swallowed, and substances that might cause infections or inflammation (aka antigens). Last but not least, it also moonlights as part of many other regulatory, metabolic, and immunity-related functions that affect the whole body.

Your Amazing Gut

The immune system in your gut is special, and it is called the gut-associated lymphoid tissue (GALT). The GALT is a gatekeeper. What makes it special is that the GALT not only knows to protect the rest of the body from microorganisms and toxins that might make you sick, but it also knows when it should allow nutrients to move from inside the digestive tract across the border into the bloodstream without triggering the immune alarm system. It continues to use its gatekeeper skills in the large intestine, where the GALT must recognize and welcome more than a trillion (10^{12} to 10^{14}) regular residents (the harmless bacteria in your gut called the gut microflora or gut microbiota), which in turn help fight off any invading (possibly harmful) bacteria that don't belong in the neighborhood.

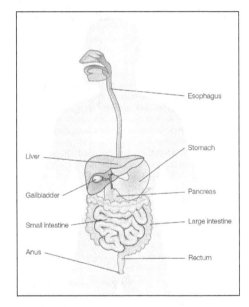

The GALT Remembers All of Its First Dates

As foods get introduced to the new gut in infancy and later, the immune system does some initial stock-taking and basically creates a special tag for foods it decides are safe. These tags are shared with the GALT, so that the next time it encounters this food, it doesn't have to take stock or evaluate it because it's already decided this food is OK. Consequently, the food moves through the body without incident.

When Do Things Go Wrong?

With food allergies, it's possible that the special tags are never made for the trigger food in question. Instead, the food is miscategorized as harmful, and the immune system goes to work against a harmless (and even nutritious) food. With food intolerances, things can go wrong in many ways anywhere along the digestive tract, from the body not being able to break food down into small enough pieces (e.g., missing enzymes) to the intestinal muscle not flexing its muscle the way it should (e.g., mechanical failure).

CHAPTER 3

Why Modern Testing Can't Tell Us Everything

There are several modern tests for food sensitivities, each with its strengths and its limitations.

Blood Test

Blood work can often tell us the answer to the exact question we ask of it. Does the blood contain IgE-type antibodies to dairy? Blood work can tell us yes or no. If that were all we wanted to know, that would be fine. But we also want to know if having antibodies to dairy means that eating dairy will cause symptoms, such as hives, itching, or difficulty breathing, or do other damage to the body that can't be perceived. Simply having antibodies to dairy suggests that the body is primed to react to it, but there is such a thing as a false positive. This means that antibodies to dairy are in the blood but that there are no clinical symptoms when the patient eats dairy. With the blood test alone, the patient might think he or she is not allowed to have dairy ever again, which is tough because dairy is in so many foods in the United States.

Blood tests might be a better option than skin tests if hives or eczema makes it hard to see the results of skin testing, or if medications (e.g., antihistamines or some antidepressants) might be preventing the patient from having a reaction to a food even when the patient is indeed allergic to it. Also, if the patient has ever had a severe allergic reaction (anaphylaxis), then blood testing can be safer. Or if the patient has tested positive on many skin tests for food allergies, the blood test can help confirm which foods the patient is allergic to.

Skin Test

Skin testing is another common way to test for allergies. A drop of a potential allergen is placed on the skin, and then needle pricks are used to allow the potential allergen to enter the skin. With a positive reaction, the skin develops a raised, red, itchy area. A larger red bump means it's more likely that the person is allergic. Usually, a positive test produces a red bump at least ⅛ inch larger than a control area of the skin.

If the test is negative, but the allergen being tested is still high on the suspect list, a deeper skin test can be done. This is called an intradermal skin test, in which potential allergen is injected into the skin. This test is more sensitive, and consequently produces more false positives (people test positive but then don't have symptoms caused by the suspected allergen).

Finally, there is a different kind of skin test for delayed reactions. Skin patch tests are left on for one to three days to test for conditions that take longer to cause a reaction, such as contact dermatitis. They can suggest a possible allergy, but are more useful for contact food allergies (as opposed to allergies caused by eating a food). As with the other test methods, the patch test has limitations, and may result in both false negatives and false positives, which is why it often takes more than one test to get to a reliable diagnosis. For example, a diagnosis might be made when there is a positive test result relating to a suspect food, combined with a drop in symptoms after eliminating said suspect food from the diet.

Skin Test or Blood Test?

Skin tests are more sensitive than blood tests, so a patient can have a positive skin test and a negative blood test. But both tests can be overly sensitive, resulting in many false positives, which in turn can lead to forcing patients to avoid foods when there's no reason to.

Although a skin test, a blood test, or a combination can help identify some allergies, these tests can't confirm a food allergy. Further evaluation with an elimination diet can. A diagnosis for food allergies often involves a health care professional completing a thorough medical history and then administering skin tests, blood tests, or both. It also often involves the patient keeping a food and symptom tracker and then undergoing an elimination diet and challenge.

Oral Food Challenge

One other test is the oral food challenge. If there is a possibility of a severe reaction (e.g., anaphylaxis), this test should be done only under medical supervision. The idea is to expose a patient to the food that is a suspected allergen and wait to see what happens. The initial dose is small, and the patient is observed for any reactions. Assuming all is clear, the cycle repeats, with the patient eating a little more of the food each time. These tests can be done openly, single-blinded, or double-blinded. An open test means that both patient and physician know what potential allergen is being tested. In a single-blind test, the physician knows what the patient is receiving, but the patient does not. In a double-blind food challenge, neither the physician nor the patient knows which sample the patient is getting (allergen or placebo).

The double-blind test is considered the highest quality because it removes possible bias, but it can be expensive and inconvenient.

Testing for Food Intolerances

If your food sensitivity is not an immune response, none of the allergy testing previously described is going to help, except perhaps to rule out allergies as the cause of the symptoms. Food intolerances can have different causes, including functional issues (e.g., missing enzymes), reactions to the chemical components of foods (e.g., additives), or structural issues (e.g., the digestive system doesn't move the way it's supposed to). More people suffer from food intolerances than they do true allergies (though for allergy sufferers, there is a greater chance of a severe reaction, such as anaphylaxis).

Tests for food intolerances differ according to the underlying cause of the condition. Unfortunately, although evidence of food intolerances shows up as bothersome symptoms, the ways in which many of them work are not fully understood. There are, of course, exceptions. For lactose intolerance, a breath test can be given to test for byproducts of undigested sugars (extra hydrogen). This is a good indication of an undigested sugar, such as lactose, but it is also a good indication of any kind of undigested sugar (e.g., fructose). To make the test more accurate, the patient can take the test after fasting and then having only lactose. There are about six different methods of testing for lactose, from Breathalyzer to biopsy to elimination diet, and some combination of these can give enough of a diagnosis to help the patient make any appropriate dietary changes.

CLINICAL INSIGHTS

Expert Interview with Scott H. Sicherer, MD

Given that there is no perfect one-size-fits-all test effective for diagnosing food allergies, what is your professional opinion on what the gold standard is for diagnosing food allergies?

A food allergy is an adverse health effect arising from a specific immune response that occurs reproducibly on exposure to a given food. It can usually be diagnosed with a combination of a careful medical history and supporting tests, such as allergy skin tests and/or blood tests. Both of these tests measure a protein made by the immune system that recognizes the food and tells the immune system to respond. The medical history and these tests are not perfect for a variety of reasons. The simple skin and blood tests are not fully informative because it is possible to have positive tests but tolerate the food. And it is possible to have negative tests but a true allergy where cells in the immune system are attacking proteins, and these cells are not measured by the available tests. Therefore, a medically supervised feeding of the food (food challenge) may be needed to confirm or refute a possible food allergy. When this feeding test is performed in a double-blind, placebo-controlled manner (food is hidden in another food, and the person tested is sometimes fed the real thing, sometimes not, and neither the patient nor the doctor knows which or when until the tests are over), it is considered the gold standard because biases in interpreting the results are reduced.

Food allergies involve the immune system, but food intolerances do not. How would your approach to diagnosis change for food intolerances?

For some food intolerances—nonimmune-adverse reactions—there are tests, such as breath hydrogen or evaluation of biopsies. Often the diagnosis is related to elimination of a suspected offender (e.g., lactose), watching for improvement, and then seeing if reintroduction results in the return of expected symptoms (e.g., in this case, gas, bloating, or loose stools).

Got it. So in both food allergies and food intolerances, sometimes a food elimination period and challenge can help with diagnosis. Are there other reasons an allergist would recommend an elimination diet for patients?

You need to consider diagnostics versus treatment. If I diagnose a specific allergy, then elimination is treatment. If you are allergic to peanut, avoiding it is treatment. If I have a patient with chronic allergic disease, for example, eosinophilic esophagitis (allergic inflammation of the tube connecting the mouth to the stomach) or severe atopic dermatitis (allergic eczema), I may use my knowledge of epidemiology (the common food triggers) and also results of history and testing to focus on a small set of foods to eliminate as a trial to see if symptoms improve.

This would be related to diagnosis until I "prove" whether any specific food is an issue. For example, I may have the patient off milk, wheat, and egg for two weeks to see if there are changes in the symptoms. Food challenges may be used to trial back the foods.

Scott H. Sicherer, MD, is professor of pediatrics and a researcher at the Jaffe Food Allergy Institute at Mount Sinai in New York and author of Food Allergies: A Complete Guide to Eating When Your Life Depends on It *(Baltimore: Johns Hopkins University Press, 2013).*

PART TWO
Food Allergies and Intolerances

CHAPTER 4

Frequently Asked Questions

The study of food allergies and intolerances is an active and ongoing area of research, and it grows with each passing year. This means that the understanding of food sensitivities continues to grow, but it also indicates that there are many questions still unanswered or without clear answers. This chapter provides a basic overview of how food sensitivities work and points out what is still unknown.

Q. What are the most common food allergies?
A. In children, the most common food allergies are to cow's milk, chicken eggs, peanuts, tree nuts, soy, and wheat. Interestingly, children often outgrow allergies to milk, eggs, wheat, and soy in early childhood.

In adults, the most common food allergies are to peanuts, tree nuts, fish, crustaceans (e.g., shrimp, crab, or lobster), mollusks (e.g., clams, oysters, or mussels), fruits, and vegetables.

Q. Are food allergies different from food intolerances?
A. Yes, they are. However, they can both be described as food sensitivities or adverse food reactions. Sometimes they even cause similar symptoms, such as nausea, vomiting, diarrhea, or stomach pain. Some symptoms are more typical of an allergy, and some are more typical of a food intolerance. Most health professionals agree that the defining difference is that a food allergy is the result of an abnormal immune system reaction to food, whereas an intolerance is caused by something other than an immune response.

Q. What is a food allergy?
A. A food allergy is the result of a confused immune system. Normally, we appreciate how the immune system goes to battle for us, deploying an array of defensive compounds to fight inflammation, infection, disease, and injury. It does this by recognizing and attacking substances that are foreign and harmful. When the immune system mistakenly targets a safe food, the reaction is called a food allergy.

Q. Can I have an allergy to something that is not a protein?

A. You may have heard that true allergies can be caused only by proteins. As far as we know today, this is true. That's probably because the immune system is able to detect specific proteins and interact with them. In the case of a specific allergic reaction, the immune system overreacts to specific proteins.

There are a couple of important things to keep in mind. First, proteins are abundant in many foods, from kale to chicken, not just meat or beans. In fact, there are proteins in just about all food. Second, some substances that are not proteins (e.g., nickel) are allergens. How can this be? Well, nickel in particular comes into contact with skin and binds with a protein in the skin to create a nickel-protein complex; that combination is what sets off the allergic reaction. So in the end it is still a protein that is involved in the allergic reaction.

To add one more layer to this story, it is thought that proteins must have certain characteristics to be potential allergens. Because most of us eat hundreds of millions of protein molecules a day, this is actually very good news. Only some of them have the potential to be allergens, and only some people are sensitive to them. Potential allergens are water soluble, meaning they can travel in steam and hang out in liquids. They have to be strong enough to withstand heat and acid, which means you can't cook or marinate your way around an allergen (and neither can the temperature of the stomach acids in your digestive tract). They also must have a certain size and shape of molecule to interact with the antibodies that trigger the immune response.

CLINICAL INSIGHTS

Expert Interview with Scott H. Sicherer, MD

Why are allergies specifically triggered by proteins versus other substances?

Most true allergies (food or environmental) are attributed to an immune response to proteins, rather than fats or sugars. Proteins are chains of amino acids and have diverse and unique "fingerprints" that the immune system is poised to detect. The immune system has to fight foreign invaders it has never seen previously, so it is ready to look at the unique signatures of many potential invaders. Evolution favored the detection of the unique proteins that distinguish many different potential invaders. The immune system also sees nonprotein structures that are often shared among bacteria, parasites, and viruses, but not with the same detail as with proteins.

Scott H. Sicherer, MD, is professor of pediatrics and a researcher at the Jaffe Food Allergy Institute at Mount Sinai in New York. He is author of Food Allergies: A Complete Guide to Eating When Your Life Depends on It *(Baltimore: Johns Hopkins University Press, 2013).*

Q. What is a food intolerance?

A. When eating a certain food leads to negative symptoms and the immune system is out of the picture, that is a food intolerance. Many food intolerances are the result of something going wrong during the digestion process or even after absorption, and many of the symptoms are gut-related (e.g., nausea, vomiting, and diarrhea). The immune system is not to blame in this case. Often symptoms are the result of you eating more than your personal threshold for an "offending" or "trigger" food, whether it's just a little or a lot of a specific food.

Q. Can symptoms of food intolerance actually be signs of other conditions?

A. Yes, other conditions that affect the digestive system can have symptoms similar to those of a food intolerance. For example, inflammatory bowel disease (IBD, which includes Crohn's disease and ulcerative colitis) and irritable bowel syndrome (IBS) can both have symptoms similar to those of a food intolerance to lactose. Celiac disease may also cause symptoms similar to those of a food intolerance.

Q. Could I feel symptoms after eating a food without it being either an intolerance or an allergy?

A. Yes, of course. For example, if you ate ten pizzas in twenty-three minutes, there's a pretty good chance you'd be feeling some side effects. That's not the kind of food intolerance we're talking about. Also, if you eat a bad oyster or tainted lettuce and end up with nausea, stomach cramps, and vomiting, that is food poisoning. These negative outcomes can happen to just about anyone. The hallmark of a food allergy or intolerance is that it affects only people who are specifically sensitive to a given food. Their reaction to their personal trigger food is different from what the majority of people would experience after eating the same food.

Q. How do food intolerances work?

A. Let me count the ways! First, we don't understand everything about the process of intolerances. The good news is that we can use what we do know to help people feel better. It's one of the reasons nutrition is such an exciting field; we have a lot of exploring and discovering to do. But because we don't understand food intolerances perfectly, and because there are so many ways in which the body can react poorly to a food, food intolerances can be difficult to treat. This is a prime reason for using the elimination diet.

Still, we do know a few things. We know that food intolerances are dose dependent. This means that the higher the "dose" of a food you eat, the worse your symptoms will be. We know that some intolerances occur because the body is missing an enzyme or doesn't have enough of an enzyme it needs to digest something. A good example of this is lactose intolerance; the body does not have enough of the enzyme lactase to digest the milk sugar called lactose (e.g., in milk, yogurt, and ice cream), resulting in gastrointestinal distress. Some intolerances are a reaction to druglike chemicals in certain foods and food additives, such as histamines (e.g., in alcohol, vinegars, and some artificial colors). Last, some intolerances are common enough that we can identify them when we see them; however, we don't have full knowledge of how they work. Examples of intolerances of food components include reactions to certain additives, such as sulfites, benzoates, or monosodium glutamate (MSG). Sulfites can be found in wine and some dried fruits; benzoates are in some preservatives and cinnamon; and MSG is sometimes added to foods or can be found naturally in some foods, such as tomatoes and mushrooms.

Q. What about food tolerance? How does it work?

A. It's easy to take "food tolerance" for granted because it is the body's normal state, and it is unremarkable because food tolerance doesn't have the uncomfortable side effects of food intolerance.

Current scientific opinion suggests that under normal conditions, the body learns to tolerate foods in infancy, even though foods are foreign substances. The body tests each food as it is introduced to the young immune system. In the normal scenario, new foods are tested by the immune system and recognized as safe, after which "memory cells" take up residence in the digestive tract so that it will remember that a food is safe the next time it shows up.

Q. What is an offending food? What is a trigger food?

A. These are ways of describing a food that causes negative symptoms. Although a food may be safe and even beneficial for most people, for those with food sensitivities—be they allergies or intolerances—these foods cause negative symptoms and are called trigger foods, aka offending foods. For example, a strawberry is a sweet reminder of the early days of summer for most. But if it's a trigger food for you, it probably looks more like poison. In the case of allergies, the trigger food is also called an allergen.

Q. Why is it that my sister can enjoy ice cream, but I can't go near it without getting a stomachache?

A. When it comes to food sensitivities, we don't know exactly why reactions to a certain food will differ from one person to the next, even among people in the same family. What we do know is that any food can trigger a reaction in the immune system of someone who is specifically susceptible to it, whether the person is allergic to the food or his or her body is unable to digest or absorb the food normally.

Genetics may play a role in how likely you are to develop an allergy, but it's not specific. In other words, if your mother or father is allergic to peanuts, you may inherit the tendency to be allergic but not necessarily to peanuts. You might find yourself allergic to, say, bananas.

How you first met a food can also have an effect. Did you meet it too early in life? Too late? The microbiota in the gut may also be involved, but this is an early and emerging area of science. However, it seems that the microorganisms that colonize the digestive tract can have a huge impact on how you process food. Lastly, any medications you're taking can play a role, perhaps partly because it can change your microbiota.

Q. What are some of the symptoms of a food allergy?

A. Food allergies can announce themselves in many ways. Some examples of more common symptoms are hives, eczema, stomach pain, diarrhea, nausea, vomiting, asthma, congestion, runny nose, and earache. In severe cases, the entire body reacts against a food; this is called anaphylaxis and it can be deadly.

Q. What happens during an allergic reaction to food?

A. The allergic reaction starts with an allergen, a food protein that triggers an allergic reaction in someone who is specifically sensitive to it. The allergen enters the body, and the immune system goes to work: Its white blood cells (leukocytes) go into defensive mode and release chemicals that under normal circumstances are meant to protect the body, but they also cause the negative symptoms of an allergy.

Imagine your immune system is a 911 emergency call center. In an allergic reaction, the allergen is like the phone call to the call center that sets everything else in motion. The operator in charge of your case is like the type of white blood cells called the T-helper cells. They are in charge and will manage the rest of what's about to happen, including dispatching emergency responders, such as police or an ambulance. In the immune response, the emergency responders, called cytokines, are the messenger chemicals.

Continuing with the metaphor, let's say the 911 operator responds to two kinds of calls on a typical workday. One is the common my-cat-is-up-a-tree or my-neighbor's-music-is-too-loud kind of call. The other type of call, thankfully, isn't as common: maybe someone's house is on fire or someone has fallen down the stairs. The first kind of call is like what happens in a T-helper cell reaction type 1. The second kind of call, T-helper cell reaction type 2, is like the immune reaction that happens only in people who are specifically sensitive to a given allergen. In reaction type 2, the T-helper cells include a special set of cytokines (emergency responders) in the immune response and a specific type of antibody is created called an IgE antibody. This type of antibody triggers a series of reactions that can result in symptoms typical of allergies, such as hives, hay fever, itching, swelling, reddening, and asthma.

CHAPTER 5

Common Food Allergies

Eight foods trigger about 90 percent of food allergies: milk, eggs, wheat, peanuts, soy, tree nuts, fish, and shellfish. In the United States, the eight major allergens must be listed on labels of packaged foods. This chapter covers the eight major allergens, as well as a few other foods and substances that are linked to allergies.

Milk

When we discuss a milk allergy, we are referring to an allergy to cow's milk, which contains more than twenty proteins, each of which could potentially trigger an allergic reaction. Some milk proteins are destroyed in cooking, but because it's common to be allergic to more than one protein in milk, the usual way to manage a milk allergy is to avoid it altogether. That said, goat's milk and sheep's milk allergies are more frequent in people with cow's milk allergies.

An allergy to cow's milk is the most common food allergy in infants and young children, with approximately 2.5 percent of children younger than age three allergic to milk (estimates vary; some go up to about 7 percent). Most of those with the allergy develop it in the first year of life. Interestingly, most children also outgrow a milk allergy by age four. A much smaller percentage of adults are thought to have a milk allergy (0.1 to 0.5 percent).

The amount of milk it takes to trigger an allergic reaction in someone with a milk allergy can vary from the smallest trace amounts to large volumes of milk. It all depends on the individual's threshold level. To complicate things even more, symptoms might show up just minutes after the person consumes milk or as long as a day later. Symptoms of a milk allergy range from mild (e.g., hives) to severe (anaphylaxis). The most common symptoms are related to the digestive system (bloating, pain, gas, diarrhea, constipation, nausea, or vomiting) and the skin (hives, swelling, or eczema). If the allergic person already has asthma, sometimes having milk or milk-containing foods makes it worse. Anaphylaxis is possible but rare. Further, the immune response to different proteins in milk may vary as well. This means two people who are both allergic to milk may have different sets of symptoms, making it that much harder to diagnose this kind of allergy.

Note that cow's milk allergy extends to anything with cow's milk in it, including cheeses made from it and processed foods with milk in them. This includes liquid and dry milk, yogurt, buttermilk, cheeses, ice cream, cream, butter, and many processed foods. Unfortunately, it is also a good idea to avoid goat's milk and any cheeses or other products made with it, because having a goat's milk allergy is more common in people who already have a cow's milk allergy. There is a more extensive description and list of foods to avoid in Chapter 16: How to Avoid Common Trigger Foods.

Diagnosing a Milk Allergy

An elimination diet, followed up with a food challenge, is one of the best ways to get an accurate diagnosis. A qualified allergist can also conduct a skin prick test, a blood test, or an oral food challenge (this last takes place with the patient under the allergist's supervision), but sometimes the results of these tests are conflicting. One test may show a positive result for allergies; another may have a negative result. That's why a combination of your diet history, medical history, the results of an elimination diet, and the results of the other tests mentioned in this paragraph may all help to determine the answer to the question of whether you have a milk allergy.

Milk Allergies Versus Lactose Intolerance

Both milk allergies and lactose intolerance involve negative digestive issues, such as gas, stomach pains, diarrhea, nausea, vomiting, and bloating. A milk allergy may affect other systems in the body, the way any allergy might, causing a runny nose, congestion, hives, and so on. In terms of what is going on inside the body, the milk allergy is an immune response to a protein in milk, while lactose intolerance is the body's reaction to poorly digesting and absorbing a sugar found in milk. It's possible for someone to have both, and even possible for the immune reaction to a milk allergy to cause secondary lactase deficiency. A milk allergy is much harder to manage than lactose intolerance, so it's important to figure out which one is causing your symptoms. To learn more about lactose intolerance, see "Lactose (Sugar)" section on page 63.

Getting the Nutrients Found in Milk

Milk contains many important nutrients, most of which can easily be found elsewhere, except for calcium and vitamin D, which can be more difficult. If it becomes too challenging to get these important nutrients from other foods, consider a supplement. However, there are many options for both. A cup of milk contains about 290 mg calcium (the daily recommended amount is about 1,000 mg), and any food providing 100 mg or more is considered a good source of calcium. Nonmilk foods with more than 300 mg of calcium are collard greens (1 cup), bone-in sardines (3 ounces), fortified soy milk (1 cup), tofu yogurt (1 cup), almonds (1 cup), and fortified orange juice (1 cup). Foods fortified with calcium are often fortified with vitamin D as well. The recommended daily amount of vitamin D is 600 international units (IU), which is 15 micrograms (mcg). A good source of vitamin D provides at least 10 percent of that, or 60 IU (1.5 mcg). Natural food sources of vitamin D are fish, egg yolks, and sometimes mushrooms (mushrooms exposed to UV light create their own vitamin D, and they are often labeled as a good source of vitamin D). Canned sockeye salmon has 730 IU of vitamin D in 3 ounces. A couple of scrambled eggs have 88 IU. And of course, the skin converts sunlight (UV) into vitamin D. Exposure to sunlight is a viable option if it is geographically available and done in moderation, to prevent sunburn or skin damage. A more extensive list of calcium and vitamin D foods is in the tip sheets in Chapter 15.

Eggs

Like cow's milk allergies, egg allergies are common in children younger than seven, and that is where we see the most severe reactions. In fact, the majority of food sensitivities in children younger than two comes from milk and eggs. And to be clear, when we discuss "eggs" we are referring to the common chicken egg. Egg allergies may affect 1 to 2 percent of children. As with a milk allergy, most children with an egg allergy will outgrow it. A much smaller percentage of adults are thought to have an egg allergy (0.1 percent).

Most of the proteins that trigger egg allergies are found in the egg whites. However, because it's impossible to keep the egg white from touching the egg yolk, and because some people may be sensitive to the proteins in the egg yolk (less common), people with egg allergies have to avoid eggs altogether.

Symptoms can be mild (e.g., hives) to severe (anaphylaxis, but this is rare). An egg allergy can lead to classic allergic reaction symptoms: hives, eczema, reddening, swelling, abdominal pain, nausea, vomiting, diarrhea, and hay fever–like symptoms, throat tightening, wheezing, or asthma. Raw or undercooked eggs may trigger stronger reactions than well-cooked eggs, as some of the proteins in eggs are broken down through the cooking process.

Be aware that there is a condition called food-dependent exercise-induced anaphylaxis (FDEIA), and egg allergies have been reported to trigger it. Read more about a theory of how it works in "Exercise and Allergies" on page 36. This means that eating eggs may not cause an allergic reaction in some people unless they exercise after eating them. We don't know exactly why this is so. It could have to do with exercise speeding up the body's absorption of nutrients, so that more of an allergen protein is circulating in the blood and is thus more likely to trigger an allergic reaction.

Exercise and Allergies

Where exercise is involved, food allergies are appropriately called exercise-induced food allergies. This means that it takes more than just eating a trigger food to cause an allergic reaction —exercise must be involved. If a trigger food is eaten within a couple of hours of working out, the temperature rise that happens during physical activity causes an allergic reaction. For some people, eating any food before exercise can trigger an allergic reaction, often involving itching, light-headedness, hives, and even total body shock (anaphylaxis). For others, this happens only after eating a specific food. For most people, however, there's no excuse not to eat and run.

Well, you could avoid eating for a couple of hours before exercising, but this may not be ideal if you're trying to fuel for performance or if you need to eat something during exercise, the way endurance athletes do. The most common trigger foods are crustacean shellfish (e.g., shrimp, prawn, crab, and lobster), alcohol, tomatoes, cheese, and celery. Keep a food and symptom tracker to identify potential foods to eliminate. See if the symptoms improve when you eliminate a food, and then test the food again to see if exercise induces a reaction. If all food causes a reaction, then it might indeed be a matter of avoiding eating before workouts.

http://www.niaid.nih.gov/topics/foodallergy/understanding/Pages/OASExercise-inducedFA.aspx

Egg Allergies Versus Chicken Allergies

This question is an interesting spin on the age-old question of the chicken and the egg. For the most part, an allergy to a chicken egg has nothing to do with an allergy to chicken meat. However, the chicken and the egg do have minor proteins in common, and if your body has antibodies to that exact class of proteins, then yes, you may have antibodies to both a chicken and an egg. Even in these cases, most people can eat chicken meat without symptoms. But if symptoms appear, it may be time to avoid chicken.

It may be possible to have a related reaction to eggs of other birds, including eggs from turkeys, ducks, and geese. The science is not conclusive yet, and for now chicken eggs can be thought of as completely different from other bird eggs. Still, it may be a good idea to use an abundance of caution and try a little of these nonchicken eggs first to see if there is a reaction. In the same vein (an abundance of caution), it is often recommended that children who are allergic to eggs avoid all kinds of bird eggs.

Diagnosing an Egg Allergy

A blood test can be done to see if your blood has the specific type of antibodies to eggs (IgE type) that might lead to an allergic reaction. However, this method has often resulted in false positives. In other words, though the egg antibodies are in the blood, eating eggs did not cause an allergic reaction. Another test that may be more reliable is a skin test. These tests, along with a detailed medical history and exam, followed by an elimination diet and challenge, can help diagnose an egg allergy.

Vaccines and Egg Allergies

Some medications and vaccines may contain egg or ingredients made from egg. The reason these vaccines contain egg proteins is that the viruses used in vaccines are often grown in an egg (viruses need a living host to grow on). Some of the common vaccines that may contain egg proteins include the MMR vaccine (the one for measles, mumps, and rubella) and the flu shot. Egg proteins can make their way in to other vaccines, too, so it's a good idea to ask your clinician and to let him or her know if you have an egg sensitivity. Thankfully, strong reactions to vaccines are rare. Mild or strong, reactions to vaccines are tricky because it can be hard to identify which component triggered a reaction (the vaccine antibodies, the egg protein, the gelatin, and so on).

Getting the Nutrients Found in Eggs

Eggs contain many important nutrients, most of which can easily be found elsewhere. Two nutrients in eggs that many people may not be getting enough of are vitamin D and folacin (a form of folate). Vitamin D can be found in some mushrooms (mushrooms exposed to UV light create their own vitamin D, and they are often labeled as a good source of vitamin D), seafood, and supplements. Folate can be found in spinach, beans, Brussels sprouts, enriched wheat and rice, and supplements. Other nutrients in eggs are quite easy to obtain in a varied and balanced diet that includes meat, fish, poultry, beans, whole grains, and vegetables. These are vitamin B12, pantothenic acid, the antioxidant selenium, riboflavin, biotin, iron, antioxidant vitamins A and E, vitamin B6, and zinc.

Wheat

Wheat allergies are more common in young children, though they often outgrow it by age three. Estimates of how many people have wheat allergies vary widely around the world and even within the United States. Two studies, ten years apart, from 1990 and 2000, estimate that the percentage of people with a wheat allergy ranges from 2.5 percent to 20 percent, which is an indication that diagnosis methods were very different. Still, it is one of the eight major allergens responsible for 90 percent of all allergic reactions in the United States.

Grains, such as wheat, are not the first foods that come to mind when thinking about protein. Still, wheat is about 10 percent protein, with well over fifty distinct proteins. Many of these proteins are allergenic, though specific proteins have not been singled out as the problem. There are four main types of proteins in wheat: gliadins, glutenins, albumins, and globulins. Research is under way, and at some point we may understand more about specific proteins or protein classes and how they are involved in wheat allergies. For now, we understand that a person with a wheat allergy is probably reacting to several different proteins in wheat.

Symptoms can either be immediate or slightly delayed. Immediate symptoms may start within minutes of eating wheat or up to a few hours afterward. Slightly delayed symptoms can appear one to two days after eating wheat. The symptoms vary from mild (e.g., hives) to severe (e.g., anaphylaxis). A wheat allergy can affect any organ system, including the systems for digestion, breathing, the skin, and the mouth. Digestive symptoms are the most common; they include stomach pain, diarrhea, and sometimes nausea and vomiting. Breathing difficulties include asthma and airway constriction, which can make it hard to breathe (bronchospasm). Skin symptoms include eczema, hives, and swelling, often in the face. Symptoms in and around the mouth include itchy throat and mouth, tongue irritation, swelling, burning, and throat tightness.

As with an egg allergy, a wheat allergy can be worsened by exercising. See page 36 for more information on food-dependent exercise-induced anaphylaxis.

Unfortunately the only way to avoid an allergic reaction is to avoid the trigger food. It can be difficult to avoid wheat in the United States, as it's everywhere: in our breads, cereals, pastas, crackers, cookies, and more. In the United States, wheat must be listed clearly in the ingredients statement of packaged foods, so that people with wheat allergies can clearly identify foods that are unsafe for them. Remember that wheat goes by many names:

• Bulgur	• Farro	• Spelt
• Durum	• Graham	• Sprouted wheat
• Einkorn	• Kamut	• Triticale
• Emmer	• Seitan	• Wheatberries
• Farina	• Semolina	• Wheatgrass

Check out the tip sheets for information on reading ingredients labels (page 157), hidden sources of wheat (page 184), and more.

Distinguishing Between a Wheat Allergy, Celiac Disease, and Gluten Intolerance

Squares are a special type of rectangle. All squares are rectangles. But not all rectangles are squares. Think of people with a wheat allergy as people who are not allowed to eat from square plates (wheat). Meanwhile, people with celiac disease or a gluten sensitivity have to avoid square plates (wheat) and all other rectangular-shaped plates (rye and barley), too. This is because wheat contains gluten, but not all gluten-containing foods have wheat in them. Also, a wheat allergy involves a classic allergy immune response to wheat (using IgE-type antibodies). With a gluten sensitivity, the body is reacting to a specific protein—gluten—which is found in wheat, rye, and barley. With celiac disease, the body's immune system is also involved, but it's a more specialized reaction (using IgA-type antibodies). Finally, although an allergy to wheat can trigger reactions throughout the body, a gluten sensitivity mostly triggers digestive issues. Learn more about celiac disease and gluten sensitivities in the section on celiac disease (page 74).

Diagnosing a Wheat Allergy

There are some issues with the diagnostic tests for wheat allergy. The standard practices of taking a detailed medical history and then testing skin, blood, or both for wheat-specific antibodies are a good start but can be misleading. Because a few different types of antibodies could be involved, a test that is designed to identify one may not pick up the other and vice versa. Because of this complication with wheat allergy, sometimes test results show a false negative, even though a food challenge clearly triggers symptoms. To get a clearer picture, once wheat is a suspected trigger food, it's helpful to eliminate it from the diet until symptoms lessen or clear and then reintroduce it to see if it triggers symptoms.

Getting the Nutrients Found in Wheat

In the US diet, wheat and wheat products are an important source of vitamins and minerals, including thiamine, riboflavin, niacin, iron, selenium, chromium, magnesium, folate, phosphorus, and molybdenum; some of these nutrients are added in the process of enriching foods that contain wheat. Wheat is the main grain in the US food system, but there are many other grains to enjoy.

Rice, corn, oats, and barley have always been viable alternatives to wheat. And with the growing awareness of wheat and gluten sensitivities, many other alternatives are becoming available in mainstream markets, including rye, buckwheat, amaranth, quinoa, millet, and tapioca. Some of these are enriched with some of the nutrients included in enriched wheat. If you're looking for a starch to replace wheat on the plate, potatoes, yams, sweet potatoes, and parsnips are also options.

Peanuts

The reports about how many people have peanut allergies vary from country to country. Some estimates say that the number of children in the United States with peanut allergies tripled between 1997 and 2008. Is that due to more allergies or different methods of diagnosis? The answer is unclear, but some studies indicate that about 20 percent of children with a peanut allergy outgrow it. If and when more is known about the exact mechanism of how a peanut allergy works, we can develop better ways to diagnose, treat, and maybe even prevent peanut allergies.

Peanuts are actually related to soybeans, peas, all kinds of beans, and lentils. In other words, peanuts are a legume. If you are allergic to peanuts, you have a greater chance of having a related allergy to, say, soy, as it's also in the legume family, than a tree nut. Peanuts are categorically different from tree nuts, such as almonds, walnuts, and cashews. The confusion is that peanuts are largely eaten like nuts in the United States—as a snack, as a spread, in baking, and so on. Another example of this food category confusion is tomatoes: botanically, they are a fruit, but are thought of and used in kitchens across the country as a vegetable.

The issue with tree nuts is that they may come into contact with peanuts in nut mixes, or scoops may be used to touch peanuts and then tree nuts, thereby cross-contaminating the tree nuts with peanut proteins. The same idea of cross-contamination can affect any food (e.g., candy, cookies, or ice cream) that is made with machinery that is also used with peanuts. In addition, tree nuts are also one of the eight major food allergens and can trigger strong reactions.

Thankfully, there's no evidence that people with peanut allergies need to avoid all legumes. People with peanut allergies and allergies to other legumes may simply be allergic to each food specifically, not because they are related. This is good news, as legumes are uniquely nutritious. They are excellent sources of plant protein, dietary fiber, and important nutrients, such as iron, zinc, folate, and potassium; this all means that legumes can provide some of the important nutrients found in meats, fruits, and vegetables. They can also be quite affordable and come in a variety of convenient forms (dry, canned, and frozen).

Like all food allergies, a peanut allergy can trigger reactions in many different organ systems (skin, lung, digestive, heart, and total body). And, as with all food allergies, not all people will experience the same symptoms, or even all of the symptoms, and the symptoms they do experience can range from mild to severe. That said, peanuts are well known for their potential to cause severe total-body reactions (aka anaphylaxis).

Skin symptoms include hives, reddening, and swelling. Skin symptoms often affect the face. Breathing issues include wheezing, noisy breathing, cough, difficulty breathing, throat tightening, and nasal congestion, and for those who already have asthma, it may trigger asthma. Digestive complaints include vomiting, diarrhea, and stomach pain. Your blood pressure may drop, or you may experience an irregular heart rate (a normal heart rate is about 50–100 beats per minute). In the worst-case scenario, symptoms can include anaphylaxis, a severe, whole-body allergic reaction.

The Food and Drug Administration (FDA) is, as of the writing of this book, investigating how much peanut-containing food will cause an allergic reaction. At the beginning of 2013, the FDA put out a wide request for data on what safe levels of an allergen might be, so that it can decide if it can safely establish threshold levels for major food allergens. What this means for the consumer is that if a safe level can be determined, foods that qualify can be labeled as XXX-free (e.g., "peanut-free"), probably with some level of testing to support the claim. It could potentially make it easier for people with food allergies to find foods that are safe for them. However, as of now FDA has no such regulation in place, and health professionals tend to agree that it is difficult to determine how much peanut will cause a reaction in one person versus the next. Similar to other allergies, the trigger amount could be as small as particles that are inhaled or as large as 1 gram, 10 grams, 100 grams, or 1,000 grams. Those numbers are purely for illustration, because *anyone* who eats 1,000 grams of peanuts (more than thirty-three servings!) might not feel great.

Diagnosing a Peanut Allergy

Like a diagnosis of other food allergies, figuring out if you have a peanut allergy starts with a good medical history, a food and symptom tracker, and an exam. A physician can help rule out other causes of your symptoms. If your symptoms are pointing toward a peanut allergy, skin and blood tests can be done to see if you have specific antibodies (the IgE type) to peanuts.

However, theoretically you could use a peanut oil, a fat because allergic reactions happen only when proteins are present. Highly refined oils are all fat and no protein—or so we thought. Recently, very sensitive measurement techniques were able to find extremely small amounts of peanut protein in highly refined peanut oil. Someone would have to be extremely sensitive to peanuts to react to peanut oil, but it's possible.

Getting the Nutrients Found in Peanuts

Peanuts do have vital nutrients, but these nutrients can be easily found in alternative foods in a balanced and varied diet. Some of the important nutrients are protein, healthy unsaturated fats, niacin, magnesium, vitamin E, manganese, pantothenic acid, chromium, vitamin B6, folacin, copper, and biotin. All of these nutrients are easy enough to find by eating a mix of other legumes, whole grains, vegetables, vegetable oils, and meat.

The challenge of a peanut allergy is that peanuts are used in many different foods in the US food supply, so they can be hard to avoid. In the United States, a food label has to say *peanuts* if any of the ingredients are made from peanuts.

Do note that, roasting peanuts, particularly versus boiling them, seems to make them more likely to trigger an allergic reaction. Most of the peanuts and peanut products in the United States are roasted. In other countries and other cuisines, peanuts are boiled and eaten more like legumes.

Soy

Of the many proteins in soy, studies have identified about ten of them as potential triggers for an allergic reaction. However, we don't yet have the final word on which proteins in soy are guilty. Unfortunately, we don't know a lot about how this allergy works, just that soy is definitely one of the more common triggers for a food allergy. Less than one-half percent of children are allergic to soy (0.4 percent), and it's common for them to outgrow the allergy by their third birthday. Further, the majority of children with soy allergies will outgrow them by their tenth birthday. We're not sure how many adults have soy allergies.

Symptoms are generally mild (e.g., hives), though there are rare cases of severe reactions (anaphylaxis). There are many similarities to milk allergy. The most common symptoms are related to the digestive system (bloating, pain, gas, diarrhea, constipation, nausea, vomiting, and cramping) and the skin (hives, swelling, and eczema). Breathing issues include coughing, sneezing, wheezing, congestion, and runny nose.

Soy foods are not traditionally an important part of the US diet, the way that wheat is, for example. But soy has found its way into more and more processed foods, making it hard to avoid. In addition, as the country has become more multicultural, some traditionally Asian soy-containing foods have become more common in the US diet (e.g., soy sauce, tofu, miso, edamame, and tempeh). If you have a soy allergy, avoid eating at Asian restaurants; the risk of cross-contamination with soy is high, even if you order a soy-free item. An increased interest in vegetarian and vegan diets may also contribute to the increase in soybean products, such as soy milk and soy cheese, in the marketplace. Avoiding soy means avoiding soybeans and all soy-containing foods and products.

The good news is that it's very rare to be allergic to other foods in the highly nutritious legume family just because you're allergic to soy (or peanuts). The legume family includes beans, peas, lentils, alfalfa, clover, carob, tamarind, lupins, and more. Beans and peas, in particular, are unique foods because they are part of two food groups: the protein group and the vegetable group.

Much of the vegetable oil on the market is part or all soybean oil. Pure oil is 100 percent fat, especially if it is highly refined, and most people with soy allergies can tolerate a small amount of soy oil; the FDA even exempts highly refined soybean oil from being labeled as an allergen. However, because trace amounts of soy protein could potentially be in the oil, people who are very sensitive to soy should probably avoid it and look for alternative vegetable oils. Further, cold-pressed oils are generally less refined, so a cold-pressed soybean oil is more likely to contain soy protein. Other terms for *cold-pressed* are *pure-pressed*, *expeller-pressed*, *extruded*, and *unrefined*.

Diagnosing a Soy Allergy

Your doctor will likely take a thorough medical history and do a careful exam, and he or she may do some skin or food challenge testing with you. Sometimes results from these tests do not agree, making it difficult to get a clear diagnosis. For example, test results might differ if the IgE-type antibodies are not involved in the allergic reaction. Skin tests will test for IgE antibodies. But food challenges simply test for a reaction to eating a food.

Getting the Nutrients Found in Soy

Soybeans themselves are a good source of protein, and they also provide B vitamins, such as thiamine, riboflavin, vitamin B6, and folacin, as well as minerals, such as phosphorus, magnesium, iron, calcium, and zinc. Look to other legumes, particularly beans and peas, to get some of the same nutrients. Soy-containing processed foods usually don't have significant amounts of nutrients from soy, so there is less of a nutritional loss in avoiding those sources of soy in the US food supply.

Tree Nuts

There is not a huge amount of information on how many people are affected by tree nut allergies. However, the US estimate is 0.5 percent of the population, or about 1.5 million people. In various countries in Europe and the Middle East, estimates vary from .03 percent (Israel, about 24,000 people) to 8.5 percent (Germany, about 6.9 million people). In the United States, because the need and the risk is relatively high, the presence of tree nuts in a food must be declared on the label. Because most people don't think of specific nuts as "tree nuts," the label is required to name the specific nut it contains. This is because tree nuts are relatively common among food allergens, and they can trigger a whole-body (anaphylactic) reaction. It used to be thought that a tree nut allergy was an allergy for life, but recent studies suggest that 9 percent of children with tree nut allergies outgrow the condition. Of course, being allergic to more than one tree nut makes it more likely that you'll have an allergy for life.

Tree nut allergies work in the same way most other food allergies work. The body reacts to a specific protein in the tree nut, which it mistakes as harmful, and mounts an immune system attack. Nuts and seeds may be highly allergenic because they are the reproductive part of a plant. They also contain a class of proteins that plants use as a defense mechanism during times of stress; this is often linked to food allergies.

So, what exactly is a tree nut? Most people think of the nuts themselves, e.g., almonds, walnuts, cashews, and so on, rather than the category called tree nuts. Or they think of the category called nuts. The reason there's a difference in terminology is that saying *nuts* could be confusing; a person might think of peanuts (which is a legume, not a tree nut), coconut (a fruit, not a tree nut), nutmeg (a spice, not a nut), or butternut squash (a squash, not a nut). Tree nuts grow on, well, trees. The more common tree nuts in the US diet include almonds, Brazil nuts, cashews, hazelnuts, macadamia nuts, pecans, pine nuts, pistachios, and walnuts. Interestingly, some of the tree nuts the FDA includes on their "must be labeled" list are not known to cause allergic reactions, and some actually aren't even nuts. See what the FDA calls a tree nut on page 45.

From a culinary perspective, tree nuts are all nuts. However, botanically speaking, they are not. In botany, a nut is the fruit and seed of plant that remains inside a hard shell (e.g., beechnuts, chestnuts, hazelnuts, acorns). Some tree nuts are technically edible seeds of a certain kind of fruit (i.e., a drupe fruit), such as almonds, pecans, pistachios, and walnuts. And there are also tree nuts that are seeds of sorts (Brazil nuts are capsule seeds, cashews are seeds of an accessory fruit, macadamia nuts are the seeds or kernels of a follicle fruit, and pine nuts are pine tree seeds. The fact that "tree nuts" have so many different origins reveals that they are not all related, and so being allergic to one does not mean being allergic to all of them. That said, an allergy to all of them does occur (but rarely) for some individuals.

In an abundance of caution, people known to be allergic to one nut are often told to avoid all nuts, but this is more to prevent contact with a cross-contaminated food than to keep them from all other nuts. For example, if you are allergic to walnuts, you would want to avoid mixed nuts, as they have come into contact with walnuts. Similarly, you'd want to avoid a muffin that was made using the same equipment that was used with walnuts.

An allergic reaction to tree nuts can affect the mouth, skin, breathing, digestion, and even the entire body's system (anaphylaxis), which can be dangerous. In and around the mouth, symptoms include tingling lips; itchy mouth, ears, and eyes; and tightening of the throat. For the skin, symptoms include hives, swelling, and pinkeye (usually from touching the trigger food and then touching the eyes). Asthma can flare up for people with asthma. The digestive system can react with stomach pain, diarrhea, or vomiting.

Diagnosing a Tree Nut Allergy

As with any diagnosis process, you'll start with a medical history and exam. Then your doctor may use skin prick and blood tests to see if you carry antibodies for nuts and seeds in general. If your test results come back positive, your doctor will follow up with tests for specific nuts and seeds. However, these methods aren't always 100 percent accurate, and there have been inconsistencies between positive blood test results and symptoms. This means that blood tests can suggest that someone has an allergy to nuts, when in reality he or she can eat them without an allergic reaction. A direct challenge with a trigger food, under medical supervision, is a better way to clearly confirm the food allergy. Because there is a risk of a severe reaction, it is important to have careful medical supervision.

FDA List of Tree Nuts

Almond

Beechnut: Technically edible but bitter. Not known to cause an allergic reaction.

Brazil nut

Butternut: A native American nut, dubbed the white walnut; is not related to butternut squash. Not known to cause an allergic reaction.

Cashew

Chestnut (Chinese, American, European, and Seguin)

Chinquapin: Similar to chestnut but smaller; not to be confused with the freshwater fish of the same name. Not known to cause an allergic reaction.

Coconut: A fruit, not a nut, but sometimes people have allergies to coconut. Still, a coconut allergy does not seem to be related to a tree nut allergy. Most people who are allergic to tree nuts can safely eat coconut. Not known to cause a tree nut allergic reaction.

Gingko nut (misspelled on the FDA website as ginko): This nut is native to China, is delicately sweet, and is in season during the fall and winter in many gourmet and Asian markets. Not known to cause an allergic reaction.

Hazelnut (aka filbert)

Heartnut

Hickory nut: Related to the pecan, which is one of the seventeen varieties of hickory nut. The common hickory nut has a very hard shell and a high fat content; it can be substituted for pecans in most recipes. Not known to cause an allergic reaction.

Lichee nut (alternative spellings are litchi, lychee, and lichi): The presence of lichee fruit on FDA's list of tree nuts is truly an oddity. It is a fruit with a perfumed, delicately sweet white flesh similar to a large grape. Originally from China, when lichees were first available in the United States it was in their dried form only, and their dry peel made them look like nuts. Dried lichee fruit tastes a little like raisins, and is a far cry from the vanilla-sweet aromas of the fresh fruit. Not known to cause an allergic reaction.

Macadamia nut (aka bush nut)

Pecan

Pine nut (aka piñon, pignoli, and pignolia): Not known to cause an allergic reaction.

Pistachio

Shea nut: Not known to cause an allergic reaction.

Walnut (English, Persian, black, Japanese, and California)

Getting the Nutrients Found in Tree Nuts

Tree nuts are one of the healthiest foods nature has provided us, which is why they are studied for their benefits in preventing and treating major chronic diseases, namely, heart disease, diabetes, and obesity. Specific nuts provide different nutrients, but most provide healthy unsaturated fats, protein, fiber, and phytonutrients. There are other food sources for all these nutrients, but if it is possible to identify the tree nuts that you are able to eat without a negative reaction, nuts are a nutrient-rich food to include in your diet. In particular, pistachios, almonds, and walnuts are great choices.

Fish

This is one food allergy that is more common in adults than in children. A 2004 study done in the United States found that 2.8 percent of adults had a seafood allergy, compared with 0.6 percent of children. About 40 percent of people with a fish allergy have their first allergic reaction as adults. If you're allergic to one type of fish, there's a more than 50 percent chance that you'll be allergic to another type of fish.

A fish allergy actually refers to fin fish, which are free-swimming fish, such as tuna, salmon, trout, cod, sole, catfish, halibut, mackerel, pollock, sea bass, and so on. Shrimp and oysters are in a category of seafood called shellfish, which is quite different from fin fish. That said, some people with a fin fish allergy may also have a shellfish allergy. For more on what it means to have a shellfish allergy, see page 48.

There is a lot we don't know about fish allergens, except for one specific class of allergens protein called parvalbumins, which were originally found in cod. They can actually be found in a variety of fish that aren't even related to cod. Currently, we think the majority of fish allergies may be related to parvalbumins, rather than the proteins that might be specific to a certain fish. But because we don't know for sure, and because fish are such a nutrient-rich food that most people should include more of in their diets, the best-case scenario is to avoid only the fish you know you're allergic to. The exception to this is when you know you may have an anaphylactic reaction, in which case, in an abundance of caution, it may be best to avoid fish altogether.

Parvalbumins are found in the muscle of fish, are water soluble (so fish stews will have the proteins in the liquid, as will the steam from a fish dish), are heat resistant (so cooking won't destroy them), and are generally resilient. More than fifty fish species are known to contain parvalbumins, including cod, tuna, anchovy, perch, mackerel, sardines, salmon, flounder, catfish, tilapia, eel, herring, carp, sea bream, and more.

Who Knew? Beer and Wine May Contain Trace Amounts of Fish

First, keep in mind that the risk of an allergic reaction to beer or wine with trace amounts of fish is very low, but for those who are extremely sensitive, this may be of interest.

Some wines and beers use a fish-derived product called isinglass as part of their clarifying process. It gently clears any remaining yeast and solids out of the final product without affecting flavor. It is a traditional practice in the making of beer and wine, dating back centuries. Although isinglass is not purposely part of the final product, there is always the chance that there are trace amounts.

An online vegan guide to beer, wine, and liquor provides a simple green or red coding system, identifying products as vegan-friendly or not-vegan-friendly. Guide editors contact producers and post the producers' replies about the vegan status of their products, which sometimes indicate that they use a fish-derived product in their processing. However, the guide doesn't always specify whether a producer uses isinglass, and the not-vegan-friendly products could also include those that use, for example, egg whites in the processing. Contacting a producer directly is always a good idea, but this website may be a good first place to look. The website includes contact information for the producers: www.barnivore.com.

Fish allergies can cause severe reactions (anaphylaxis), with the most common culprits being salmon, tuna, and halibut. Other symptoms include diarrhea, nausea, vomiting, asthma, congestion, hives, itching, overall swelling, and swelling in particular of the lips and tongue. Reactions are triggered by eating fish but also by breathing in its steam, which can carry proteins in it.

Fish can potentially show up in Caesar salad dressing, Worcestershire sauce, bouillabaisse, imitation fish or shellfish, meatloaf, barbecue sauce, sausage, flavorings, or even in some trace amounts in beer and wine.

Fish oil supplements are popular for their omega-3 content, and although pure oil is 100 percent fat, especially if it is highly refined, there is the possibility that fish oils contain some trace amounts of fish protein. People who are allergic to fish are usually advised to avoid fish oil, especially if there is a risk of a severe reaction, such as anaphylaxis. There are vegetarian sources of omega-3s, which are derived from sea algae.

Diagnosing a Fish Allergy

As with any diagnosis process, you'll start with a medical history and exam, and then your doctor may use skin prick and blood tests to see if you carry antibodies for fish. If your test results come back positive, your doctor will follow up with tests for specific fish.

Getting the Nutrients Found in Fish

Fish is a nutrient-rich food that most Americans should be eating more of. Notably, some fish provide omega-3 fatty acids, and fish generally provide B vitamins, such as niacin, vitamin B6, and vitamin B12, as well as vitamins A and E, plus phosphorus, selenium, magnesium, iron, and zinc. Some fish provide vitamin D and calcium as well.

Shellfish

One survey of nearly 15,000 people in the United States found that about 2 percent of people had a shellfish allergy. Shellfish allergies are more likely to be lifelong, and they affect more adults than children. In fact, shellfish allergies are the number one food allergy of adults in the United States. About 60 percent of people with a shellfish allergy have their first allergic reaction as adults. The most common trigger foods are shrimp, crab, and lobster.

Though it's always possible you are allergic to both shellfish and fish, it is unlikely. Shellfish and fish (fin fish) are from unrelated families, even though we think of both as seafood. Within the shellfish category, there are crustacean shellfish and mollusk shellfish. The crustacean group includes shrimp, prawns, scampi, crab, lobster, and crayfish. The mollusk shellfish group includes oysters, mussels, scallops, clams, snails (e.g., escargots), abalone, squid (e.g., calamari), and octopus. For more information on fin fish allergies, see page 46.

There is a lot we don't know about shellfish allergens, but we do know about one specific allergen protein called tropomyosin, which can be found in shrimp, lobster, crab, squid, oyster, snail, mussels, clams, and scallops. It's found in the muscle meat of these shellfish, and it has also been found in the cooking water used to boil them. People who are allergic to shellfish may have antibodies to tropomyosin, and coming into contact with it will trigger the allergic reaction sequence.

Shellfish allergies can cause severe reactions (anaphylaxis), with the most common trigger foods being shrimp, crab, and lobster. Reactions to crustacean shellfish tend to be severe. Other symptoms include diarrhea, nausea, vomiting, asthma, congestion, hives, itching, overall swelling, and swelling in particular of the lips and tongue. Reactions are triggered by eating shellfish but also by breathing in its steam, which can carry proteins in it.

Diagnosing a Shellfish Allergy

As with any diagnosis process, you'll start with a medical history and exam, and then your doctor may use skin prick and blood tests to see if you carry antibodies for shellfish in general. If your test results come back positive, your doctor may follow up with tests for specific shellfish. Or your doctor may stop there, because having a shellfish allergy of any type makes it more likely for a person to be sensitive to any other type of shellfish, even unrelated species (e.g., you may be told to avoid octopus when your allergy is to shrimp). If you are allergic to one type of shellfish, you may potentially be able to enjoy shellfish from the other group, though you'll want to check with your doctor first. Because most people who are allergic to shellfish are allergic to more than one, most people are advised to avoid all shellfish.

Getting the Nutrients Found in Shellfish

Shellfish are a great lean protein source and provide potassium, zinc, selenium, iodine, and iron, as well as important B vitamins. They also provide omega-3 fatty acids, though less than fatty fin fish, such as salmon and herring. Many of these nutrients can be found in other foods, including vegetarian omega-3 supplements, derived from sea algae. One form of omega-3 fats can also be found in walnuts.

Nickel

This one is interesting. Nickel falls in a category of substances called haptens, which are small molecules that, when combined with proteins, can spark the production of antibodies that bind specifically to these molecules. Where there are antibodies, there is the possibility of an immune system reaction. Although nickel is not a protein, it binds with proteins that already exist in the body, and that combination can trigger an allergic reaction. There are educational video clips online about the process, and it's OK not to know all the chemistry they talk about; you'll still get a sense of what is happening.

Nickel is surprisingly common in our food system. It is naturally found in some foods, but it can also get into foods through industrial processing and at-home cooking. In terms of natural sources, the amount of nickel in a plant food depends on the amount in its soil, which can be affected by the season: Plants have more nickel in the spring and fall and less in the summer. Nickel also varies depending on the part of the plant; for example, there is more nickel in the leaves of a plant than in the stem or root. Further, older leaves tend to contain more nickel.

The amount of nickel in seafood depends on the amount in its environment, whether ocean, river, sea, or some other watery habitat. Nickel also finds its way into food during processing. Imagine wheat being turned into flour via metal grinders. This contact with metal can transfer some nickel into the flour. At home, when foods are cooked in stainless steel pots and pans or eaten with stainless steel utensils, nickel can be transferred into foods.

There are studies that show a nickel deficiency can have an effect on growth and development, and that nickel may do the body some good by participating as a cofactor in normal biological processes. However, the evidence doesn't give us a clear picture of how nickel works to keep us healthy. One study suggests that 25–35 mcg per day is enough, but there is not enough data to have a recommended amount of dietary nickel per day. We do, however, have an upper limit: 1 mg per day (1 mg–1,000 mcg) for adults. US adults take in an average of 100 mcg on the high end, so it seems that overdoing it on nickel through the diet is very rare. It's more common to get higher levels of nickel from dietary supplements, not food. In countries where they eat more vegetables and whole grains than Americans typically do, the nickel intake is higher but still less than the limit of 1 mg per day. Of course, the safe upper limits for nickel intake apply to the general population. People who are sensitive to nickel will want to keep their intake on the low end anyway.

All of this means that a nickel-free diet is virtually impossible, but keeping dietary nickel low might mean fewer and milder flare-ups. The key is to avoid foods high in nickel. Nickel isn't currently reported in the United States Department of Agriculture (USDA) nutrient database, perhaps because nickel content does vary so widely, so it can be challenging to know how much nickel is in foods. Instead, individual research studies have tested nickel levels. See the tip sheet in the Tools section of this book in Chapter 16 for a guide to high- and low-nickel foods, but here's a preview: the most common high-nickel foods are whole grains, cocoa and chocolate, tea, nuts, beans, and seafood.

Vitamin C, coffee, tea, and milk all make it hard for the body to absorb nickel. Though tea is typically higher in nickel, research shows the amount of nickel absorbed is dampened when nickel was consumed with tea. The exact mechanism is unknown. Pregnancy and lactation also have this effect, perhaps as a defense mechanism to keep levels of nickel down because it can potentially harm a fetus or baby. In addition, iron competes with nickel for absorption by the body, so be sure to get enough iron in your diet. If more iron is absorbed, less nickel is. In fact, having an iron deficiency (a kind of anemia) makes the body prefer nickel and absorb more of it.

The concept of what it means to go on a low-nickel diet is controversial, because the amount of nickel that will cause a reaction is different in different people. The range of nickel that sparks a reaction has ranged from 0.6 mg to 2.5 mg in people who were already sensitive to nickel. One way an elimination diet can help is that it can identify if nickel is causing your skin rashes, itchiness, or redness. Going on an elimination diet may help symptoms clear, and then when a "challenge" high-nickel food is reintroduced to the diet, if you experience a flare-up, you've identified at least one probable cause.

If you have a contact allergy to nickel, avoiding it in food may help, as it has been shown to work for some people. Other studies suggest that when a nickel-sensitive person eats nickel, the symptoms are worse at first, but then they improve over the long term. There is disagreement in the field, and we don't have a clear answer yet. The answer you get from your allergist may depend on what camp he or she is in. The only way to determine if it helps is to try it.

Diagnosing a Nickel Allergy

Nickel allergies are actually well known in dermatology circles because skin contact with nickel is known to cause itching, redness, and scaly skin in those who are sensitive to it. In general, when allergies work this way, they are called contact allergies. Common points of contact are earlobes (from earrings), stomach (from metal jean buttons), or wrists (from watch wristbands). When dermatologists saw the same symptoms in people who had not been in physical contact with nickel, they started to suspect it was the nickel in foods. They can test for contact nickel allergy with a patch that puts your skin in contact with nickel. It can take two to three days for the signs and symptoms to appear, so the patch is usually left on for that long, though your clinician will likely want to take a peek after forty-eight hours. However, if you have chronic symptoms but have not touched nickel, the way to test if you are reacting to nickel in food is through an elimination diet. After several weeks on an elimination diet, if symptoms go down, you'll test your body with a high-nickel food. If symptoms return, this is a good indication that nickel is a trigger substance for you.

Corn

This is a controversial area, and some people have discarded the idea that corn allergies even exist. Still, most allergists will admit that any food containing protein has the potential to cause an allergy, including corn. More recently, since 2000, some small studies have been done on corn allergies and, although by no means considered common, corn allergies are being taken more seriously. One survey of 4,500 people found that 2 percent of people were allergic to corn, though this information was self-reported. As with many allergies, it is difficult to find an accurate number of how many people are affected.

In double-blind tests in which people did not know whether they were eating corn, those who were sensitive to corn had relatively mild symptoms, including hives, itching, throat tightening, eczema, reddening, and abdominal pain. In addition to these more immediate effects, delayed effects include headaches, migraine, fatigue, moodiness, joint and muscle pain, and symptoms that feel like a common cold, such as runny nose, sore throat, cough, trouble breathing, and lethargy. Severe reactions, such as anaphylaxis, are always possible. Further, though rare, one study cited exercise-induced anaphylaxis due to corn (see page 36 for more on exercise and allergies).

The research in the area of corn allergies is very young, dating back only a little more than ten years. Much is still unknown. Early studies have identified a couple of different proteins that might be the trigger proteins in corn. With corn being so common in the US food system, this allergy could have major implications for anyone trying to avoid corn.

Though corn is a whole grain and has nutrients to offer, removing it from the diet does not pose a significant nutrition risk. In fact, depending on how much food with corn-containing ingredients you eat now, a corn intolerance or allergy could be a blessing in disguise, because it would automatically take a lot of processed foods and drinks out of your diet.

People with allergies differ in their individual thresholds. That said, one study found that it took a little more than a half-cup of corn to trigger an allergic reaction (100 mg). Considering that corn is in a lot of foods but at a relatively low level, this could mean that some processed foods could potentially be included each day as long as the total did not go over the 100 mg level. However, corn can be simple to avoid in a whole foods diet (a diet free of processed foods). If you're committed to eating a whole foods diet without any processed foods, then there is a shorter list of corn, foods you'll need to avoid. They include corn, popcorn, polenta, and cornmeal. Some minimally processed foods, such as cornbread and corn tortillas, are examples of foods where it's easy to tell that corn is a main ingredient.

Most people with corn allergies can tolerate a small amount of corn oil. However, because trace amounts of corn protein could potentially be in the oil as a residue, people who are very sensitive should probably avoid it and look for alternative vegetable oils. Further, cold-pressed oils are generally less refined, so a cold-pressed corn oil is more likely to contain corn protein. Other terms for *cold-pressed* are *pure-pressed, expeller-pressed, extruded,* and *unrefined.*

Corn is not one of the eight major allergens that cause 90 percent of the food allergies in the United States, so FDA does not require it to be listed on a food label, the way some other allergens are. If you are looking to avoid corn, learn where it shows up commonly in foods and keywords for ingredients that include corn, even if (especially if) *corn* is not mentioned on the label. For a list of watch words to look for in processed foods, see the Tools tip sheet in Chapter 16 on how to avoid corn.

Diagnosing a Corn Allergy

As with any diagnosis process, you'll start with a medical history and exam, and then your doctor may use skin prick and blood tests to see if you carry antibodies for corn. This should be followed up by a food challenge under a doctor's supervision. This process can be further followed up on by an elimination diet to confirm the diagnosis.

Bananas and Latex

Strange, but true—yes, you can have a latex-fruit allergy. Some people with a latex allergy have an allergic reaction to certain plant products. Latex is a natural product; it's the milky sap from rubber trees. More than ten trigger proteins have been identified in latex. Someone who has a latex-fruit allergy is first and foremost allergic to latex. Botanically unrelated plants, such as rubber trees (they produce natural rubber latex) and banana trees, can produce very similar trigger proteins. But it's not just bananas. Other natural plant foods that could potentially trigger a latex-related allergy are:

• Avocado	• Kiwifruit	• Potato
• Celery	• Mango	• Rye
• Cherry	• Melon	• Strawberry
• Chestnut	• Papaya	• Tomato
• Fig	• Peach	• Wheat
• Grape	• Pineapple	
• Hazelnut	• Plum	

The allergies are not all related to fruit, but the phenomenon was first observed with fruit, so it is still known as latex-fruit allergy or latex-fruit syndrome.

The latex part of the latex-fruit allergy is a contact allergy. This means that touching rubber gloves, breathing in the dust from the gloves, or otherwise coming into contact with something made with natural rubber—such as balloons, condoms, rubber bands, erasers, or toys—may trigger a reaction if you're allergic to latex. Contact with latex is more common in hospital and food service settings, where natural rubber latex gloves might be used.

The percentage of the population allergic to latex is on a par with the percentage of the population with celiac disease (approximately 1 percent). Hospital workers and others who use latex gloves regularly are five to ten times more likely to develop a latex allergy. Another group that could be at risk of developing latex allergies is people who undergo multiple surgeries and therefore may be getting a greater-than-average exposure to latex gloves. About half of the people with a latex allergy will also be allergic to one of the plant foods listed above, because latex and those foods have very similar proteins.

Symptoms of latex-fruit allergy range from mild to severe, including anaphylaxis. Contact with latex can trigger eczema on the hands; inflammation of the skin wherever it touches latex; swelling; itchy, watery eyes; and if you have asthma, it can bring on an attack.

Diagnosing a Latex-Fruit Allergy

First, the good news: Diagnosing a latex allergy is straightforward, involving skin tests and blood tests. The results from these tests are usually reliable, making them a good tool for diagnosis. Now for the bad news: These same skin and blood tests cannot tell you what other foods you might be allergic to as a secondary condition of having a latex allergy. This is because your antibodies are specific to latex proteins; when the body also reacts to a food with a similar protein, it's because the immune system is confused (even more than it already is by having an allergy in the first place) and is mistaking the food pro-tein for the latex protein. So then you won't have antibodies to the foods themselves unless you're independently allergic to them, which is also always a possibility. Knowing this, diagnosis can still involve skin and blood tests, but the results will be negative, while a food challenge will be positive. A food chal-lenge should be done under medical supervision because there is always a chance of anaphylaxis.

In addition to avoiding latex products, you should be aware of which fruits, vegetables, and nuts could cause a reaction due to the latex allergy. If you have a question about a certain food, it's best to do a food challenge under medical supervision. There's no reason to avoid any foods on the list if you've already enjoyed them safely. Being allergic to latex does not necessarily mean you are allergic to another plant food or that you're allergic to more than one plant food.

Hayfever and Food Allergies

Being allergic to pollen may bring seasonal discomfort and pos-sibly seasonal food allergies. It doesn't happen to everyone who is allergic to pollen, but when it does, we call it oral-allergy syn-drome or pollen–food allergy syndrome. Raw fruits and vegeta-bles are some of the main culprits. Pollen–food allergy syndrome is caused by the similarity between proteins found in certain pol-lens and certain raw fruits, vegetables, and tree nuts.

We know that the group of people who get pollen–food allergy syndrome, a subset of the people who have allergies to pollen, and that number is estimated to be about 35 million Americans. However, we don't have a good estimate for those with pollen–food allergy syndrome, because the geographical and climate variables make it hard to get an accurate count. It is unusual to see it in young children. It's more common in older children to young adults; the first time they experience a pollen–food allergic reaction, it's to a food that they've been eating for years without symptoms.

If you are allergic to birch pollen, the common trigger foods include apples, almonds, carrots, celery, cherries, hazelnuts, kiwifruit, peaches, pears, and plums. If you are allergic to grass pollen, the common trigger foods include celery, melons, oranges, peaches, and tomatoes. If you are allergic to ragweed pol-len, the common trigger foods are bananas, cucumbers, melons, sunflower seeds, and zucchini.

Where's the latex?

• Grocery store checkout belts
• Restaurants where workers use latex gloves for food preparation (call ahead to ensure your safety)
• Balloons
• Auto races, which emit tire and rubber particles
• ATM machine buttons (often made of rubber)
• Other products containing latex include the following:
• Tourniquets
• Blood pressure pads
• EKG pads
• Some adhesive bandages
• Dental devices

When someone with the condition eats a trigger food, the lips, mouth, and throat feel itchy and often tingle within minutes. For some people, it takes longer for symptoms to show up, but even then, symptoms can be felt within a half-hour. Sometimes the person's lips, tongue, and throat start to swell up, the eyes get watery and itchy, and he or she also gets a runny nose and sneezes a lot. Touching the trigger food can affect the skin that comes into contact with it. For example, if your trigger food is tomatoes and you cut one open, anywhere that the juices come into contact with your skin may start to itch, swell, or develop a rash. A systemic response that affects the whole body (anaphylaxis) is rare.

You may be in luck if you enjoy the cooked version of one of the foods you are sensitive to. Uniquely, cooking breaks down the proteins behind pollen–food allergy syndrome. For example, if apples are one of your trigger foods, you should avoid raw apples, but you can still enjoy applesauce, apple pie, or baked apples. If touching apples is problematic, it can be done with protective gloves, or can be prepared by someone else or prepared commercially.

If you are allergic to pollen, it is not necessary to avoid all the common trigger foods for pollen–food allergy syndrome. In fact, restricting the diet in any way simply adds one more challenge to eating a nutritionally adequate diet, which will help keep the body healthy. Instead, it's important to identify any foods that are indeed causing a reaction by keeping a detailed food and symptom tracker. Because most reactions are immediate, you will be able to quickly identify the trigger foods. Another option is to cook the foods that are suspected triggers, making them safe to eat even when their raw form may cause symptoms. Again, if touching a trigger food is problematic, use protective gloves in food prep, or have someone else do the prep.

Diagnosing a Pollen–Food Allergy Syndrome

For foods that cause immediate symptoms, it will be clear what those trigger foods are. When symptoms don't show up immediately, it may be harder to identify the trigger foods. In this case, keep a food and symptom tracker until you have a list of potential trigger foods. Eliminate them from the diet for a couple of weeks, and then start with the food challenges. During the challenge phase, eat or touch a small amount of a suspect food, and record the results over the following four hours. If nothing happens, double the amount of the suspect food, and monitor for a reaction over the following four hours. Repeat this cycle one or two more times until either you have a reaction or you don't. At that point, you can decide whether it's right for you to keep that food in your diet.

CHAPTER 6

Common Food Intolerances

You may encounter more confusion when you tell someone you have a food intolerance than when you mention a food allergy. Even though the reaction to food allergies can vary from a runny nose to anaphylactic shock, people still understand they need to pay attention when you tell them you have a food allergy. Remember that allergies are caused by proteins (not just what we typically consider protein—chicken, beef, or tofu—but technically, any of a number of large molecules with one or more long chains of amino acids). Proteins are found in foods as diverse as rice, strawberries, wine, cucumbers, and cookies.

Food intolerances, by contrast, can be triggered by many more substances in food, from sugars to artificial colors to additives. Although food intolerances are uncommon in general, the most common triggers include sugars (even those found in fruits and vegetables), spices, compounds found in wine (and in vinegar and in other fermented foods), artificial colors, preservatives, sulfites, and monosodium glutamate. This chapter is a guide to some of the most common food intolerances.

Sulfites (Preservatives)

Because sulfites are used in a wide range of processed foods as preservatives, they are surprisingly common in our food system. You might see sulfites on a food label as "sulfur dioxide," though they are also sometimes listed simply as "sulfites," not to be confused with sulfates, which are basically harmless. Sulfites are preservatives that can protect against salmonella, prevent browning (think of those bright orange dried apricots that would otherwise be brown), and preserve wine, among other things. We don't know exactly how it works, but we do know that people, especially if they have asthma, can experience a sensitivity to sulfites.

Some sulfites occur naturally. Usually, however, they are used as preservatives in processed foods. Sulfites are good at preserving food, and the United States has a lot of processed food in its food system. Sulfites are antimicrobial, so they can keep food from spoiling. They also prevent foods from turning brown, and consumers tend to prefer foods that don't show they are breaking down and turning brown. They are antioxidants, and can keep red meat red, shrimp and lobster flesh white. Sulfites can reduce the time it takes to make bread and keep vitamin C from vanishing (which it does very easily when it's heated or exposed to light). They are used in bleaching flour, so many baked goods may have sulfites. Some bakeries are sulfite-free.

Sulfites can also be found in fruit and vegetable products, alcoholic beverages and their nonalcoholic counterparts, sweeteners, shellfish, some condiments, snack foods, bulk foods, candies, frozen pizza dough, and pastry shells. See more in "How to Avoid Sulfites" on page 164 for a more complete list.

Although some things are destroyed in the cooking process—some bacteria (which is good) and some vitamins (which is not as good)—sulfites remain unaffected. If you've ever been hiking and come home to find seed burrs, aka hitchhikers, on your socks, you will understand how sulfites attach themselves to other substances in foods, such as proteins, starches, and sugars. It is difficult to remove all traces of sulfites, even with washing or cooking.

Interestingly, sulfite sensitivity in people without asthma is rare. Of people with asthma, an estimated 3 to 10 percent of them are also sensitive to sulfites in food. Further, the reactions in people with asthma can affect the lungs, bringing on asthmatic symptoms, including wheezing, tightness of the chest, and difficulty breathing. Unfortunately, there's no evidence that avoiding sulfites will improve asthma.

In addition to asthma symptoms for those with asthma, other symptoms include flushing, feeling a temperature change, a drop in blood pressure, abdominal pain, nausea, vomiting, diarrhea, difficulty swallowing, dizziness, loss of consciousness, hives, swelling, rash, and even the extreme whole-body reaction known as anaphylaxis or nonimmune anaphylaxis. The difference between these last two terms is that anaphylaxis is an allergic reaction and can be easily tested for, but nonimmune anaphylaxis cannot be easily tested for. However, both have the same clinical symptoms and are equally dangerous.

There are no lab tests currently available to test for sulfite intolerance. That's because we don't fully understand how sulfite intolerance works, so we don't know exactly how to diagnose it. Unlike allergies, it doesn't involve IgE, so it won't show up on skin prick or blood tests. A challenge can be done, in which an allergist gives you more and more sulfites to swallow and monitors your lungs, your vital signs, and so on, for evidence of a sulfite intolerance.

There are a few theories about how sulfite sensitivities work, but none is backed up by enough evidence to provide a clear answer. Sulfur dioxide might be a substance that directly irritates the lungs, which means breathing in sulfur dioxide could lead to asthma symptoms in someone who is sensitive to sulfites. Another theory is that sulfites, though not proteins on their own, join together with a protein in food to create a new allergen. Remember that allergies can be caused only by proteins. A third theory is that people with sulfite sensitivities might not have enough of an enzyme called sulfite oxidase, which normally converts sulfites to sulfates (sulfates are safe). Without enough of this enzyme, sulfites levels could rise. These are all theories; the answer is not yet clear.

If a food has more than 10 ppm (parts per million) of sulfites, they have to be listed in the ingredients. Note that the US Food and Drug Administration (FDA) banned the use of sulfites on fresh fruits and vegetables in 1986, except on fresh grapes and sliced potatoes. The FDA also keeps sulfites out of enriched flours and grains because they provide an essential B vitamin called thiamine (B1), which is destroyed by sulfites.

Sulfites could be in foods that don't have nutrition labels, such as some bulk foods, individually sold candies, and prepared foods with an ingredient that includes sulfites but whose overall sulfite level is under the 10 ppm mark.

Avoiding sulfites in foods is a way of life for those with sulfite sensitivity. However, food is not the only problem. Many medications contain sulfites, so be sure to talk to your pharmacist about your sensitivity to sulfites. It's important to talk to your pharmacist every time you get a prescription filled because medication formulations can change. In addition, plastic bags and other packaging might be sanitized with sulfites. It's possible to be exposed to sulfites when opening a bag that has been sanitized this way; be especially cautious when opening up a bag of dried fruit, as both are potential ways to expose yourself to sulfites. These sulfites might not need to be in the list of ingredients, but they could still be a concern if you're sensitive to them.

The answer to treating a sensitivity to sulfites is simple to say but can be challenging to live: Avoid them.

Benzoates (Preservatives)

Benzoates are chemicals that are used as food additives, though some are found naturally in foods. On a food label, benzoates can show up as *benzoic acid, sodium benzoate, potassium benzoate, calcium benzoate*, or a few other terms, most of which you'll be able to spot because they end in *benzoate*. Out of these, benzoic acid is the only one that also occurs naturally in foods. These foods include berries; stone fruits; citrus fruits; certain vegetables, such as pumpkin and spinach; honey; tea; and spices, such as cinnamon, nutmeg, and cloves. See more in "How to Avoid Benzoates" on page 168.

Benzoates are preservatives that prevent foods from spoiling due to bacteria. They also preserve the color of foods. They are commonly found in flavorings for drinks, ice cream, candy, gum, icing, and pie, to name a few. Some are used as emulsifiers (they keep oil and water together, as in mayonnaise). Benzoyl peroxide is used to bleach foods, such as milk, blue cheeses, lecithin, and flour. Benzoyl peroxide is converted to benzoic acid by the time the food is eaten.

For people who are sensitive to benzoates, a range of symptoms, similar to those of an allergic reaction, have been reported. Clinically, the symptoms are often the same, even though a benzoate sensitivity is not technically an allergy (it does not involve an immune system response). Symptoms include asthma, hives, swelling, nasal congestion, eczema, headaches, and skin irritation, including inflammation of the blood vessels, which can lead to red spots on the skin.

The level of benzoates that triggers a reaction varies among individuals who are sensitive to them. Because of this variability, there are no minimum limits. Instead, people who have a benzoate intolerance need to avoid all sources of benzoates, including natural sources and processed foods that contain benzoates. For the rest of the population, the FDA currently allows a maximum of 0.1 percent of the total weight of a food as benzoates, and they are generally recognized as safe for most people.

Benzyl, benzoyl, and parabens are related compounds and could also trigger reactions. People with aspirin allergies may also have a sensitivity to benzoates because of similar chemical structures.

There is no definitive lab test for dietary benzoate intolerance. If you suspect your skin is intolerant of benzoates in a product used on the skin, then a patch test can be done. Otherwise, going through all the steps of an elimination diet can help, including a food and symptom tracker, elimination period, and food challenge.

Tartrazine (Artificial Color)

The most well-known sensitivities to artificial colors are caused by tartrazine (FD&C Yellow #5, Yellow No. 5, or Yellow 5), a common artificial yellow coloring that is used worldwide in foods, cosmetics, and medications. Food colorings allowed to be used in the United States are classified as "generally recognized as safe," or GRAS. However, to help people who are sensitive to them identify them, artificial food colorings have to be listed on food labels in the United States.

Thankfully, not all food colorings are artificial. Nature provides a wide spectrum of colors, and some make their way into our modern food system. Saffron and turmeric are spices that are used to create a yellow color. Carrot oil provides orange colors. Paprika and beetroots lend their red hues to foods. Caramel (made by cooking and burning sugar) is used as a brown color. Chlorophyll, which is what makes green plants green, can also be added to color foods green. Various fruit and vegetable juices can also lend their colors to foods.

Though the exact mechanism of a tartrazine intolerance is unclear, we know that tartrazine can increase the amount of histamine in the blood. Histamine, in turn, triggers inflammation, which is responsible for many symptoms, from a runny nose to swelling and redness. Although the symptoms can look like an allergic reaction, current evidence leaves an immune response out of it.

The most common symptoms of a tartrazine intolerance are hives and asthma. For those who already have asthma, being sensitive to tartrazine may trigger asthma or make its symptoms worse. However, people who have asthma don't necessarily need to avoid tartrazine; it is people who specifically have a sensitivity to tartrazine who should avoid it. Other symptoms include hives, itching, nasal congestion and runny nose, blurred vision, migraine headaches, and purple patches on the skin. Some of the symptoms look a lot like an allergic reaction, though technically, it is not an immune response. Symptoms seem to be triggered by both eating a food with tartrazine in it or even just coming into physical contact with it.

There may be a connection between sensitivity to aspirin and tartrazine intolerance. In one study, about half of patients with an aspirin sensitivity also reacted to Yellow 5 and vice versa. Another study found that a small amount of Yellow 5 (0.22 mg) caused a reaction in 20 percent of patients who had an aspirin intolerance.

The following foods may contain tartrazine, though not all of them do. Some manufacturers do not use artificial colors. But it's important to be aware that these foods might contain tartrazine, so you should check the label:

• Bottled sauces	• Fruit punch	• Mustard
• Cake mixes	• Gelatin	• Pickles
• Candy	• Ice cream	• Salad dressing
• Chewing gum	• Instant pudding	• Smoked fish
• Colored sodas	• Jams	• Yogurt
• Dried and canned soup	• Jellies	

It varies by country, but in the United States, it will be shown on a food label as FD&C Yellow #5. In cosmetics, it might appear as Yellow 5. In medications, it might be listed as *tartrazine*. In some European countries, tartrazine is banned.

Currently, we don't have a way to test for tartrazine intolerance with a lab test the way we test for an allergy. The way to find out if you are tartrazine intolerant is to remove it from the diet—as you will if you follow the elimination diet in this book—and then reintroduce it during a challenge phase to see if it caused your symptoms. During the challenge phase, you'll need to test with greater and greater doses until you react. This is how you'll be able to determine what level is safe for you in the long run.

Once you have determined that your body reacts negatively to tartrazine, and once you know the amount it takes to trigger that reaction, design a lifelong diet that minimizes artificial colors and keeps your daily intake below your personal trigger level. A nice side effect of this approach is you might be eating fewer processed foods and eating more whole foods, including fruits, vegetables, whole grains, seafood, and nuts, which are important for a healthy diet.

Monosodium Glutamate (MSG)

MSG is a flavor enhancer that is commonly used in Asian cuisines, though it's also used in some American foods. Think of MSG in the same way you think of salt; it's used in a similar way. MSG sensitivity may affect as many as 1.8 percent of US adults. Like other foods that cause allergies and intolerances, it is generally safe for most of the population to eat. On average, Americans get 1.3–2 grams per day from natural and added sources. We don't know how an intolerance to MSG works, but there are some theories. Even if we don't understand the direct cause and effect, changing the diet can still help.

Compounds that resemble MSG are naturally found in tomatoes, mushrooms, soy sauce, and some cheeses. These natural glutamates contribute to the umami (savoriness) of these foods. Umami is one of the five basic tastes in addition to sweet, sour, salty, and bitter.

The list of processed foods that could contain MSG is considerably larger:

- Bottled and canned sauces
- Canned meats
- Canned soups
- Cookies and crackers
- Croutons
- Cured meats
- Diet foods
- Dry soup mixes
- Freeze-dried foods
- Frozen foods
- Gravy
- Mayonnaise
- Potato chips
- Prepared dinners and side dishes
- Prepared snacks
- Prepared salads
- Salad dressings
- Seasoning mixes
- Smoked meats and sausages

Symptoms of MSG sensitivity usually show up within half an hour of eating MSG, but some symptoms show up hours later. Common symptoms include headache, flushing, nausea, stomach cramps, and asthma in people who already have asthma. Many symptoms have been reported, though it's tough to confirm if they are directly related to MSG intake. Many symptoms are reportedly felt in the head, including facial flushing, facial numbness, tightness in the face and jaw, tingling and burning in the face, headache, blurred vision, seeing shining lights, and slurred speech. Other symptoms include rapid heartbeat, diarrhea, weakness, dizziness, balance problems, chills and shaking, sweating, difficulty breathing, water retention, thirst, insomnia, sleepiness, heavy arms and legs, stiffness, mood changes, irritability, depression, and paranoia. Not all symptoms will be felt at the same time, of course; these are symptoms that have been reported in studies.

In the 1990s, the United States Food and Drug Administration (FDA) asked an independent scientific group to look into how much MSG will trigger symptoms. The report found that it took 3 grams of pure MSG (without food) to cause a reaction in MSG-sensitive people, and that a person is unlikely to eat 3 grams in one sitting. The report stated that a typical serving of food with added MSG has less than 0.5 grams of MSG; remember that the average total daily intake in the United States is no more than about 2 grams.

Because there is no universal amount of MSG that will trigger symptoms, it is important to tune into your individual diet to figure out what your personal limit is. You'll have to avoid all sources of MSG, added or natural, and keep your total MSG levels below your limit. An elimination diet can help determine if MSG is causing your symptoms.

The process of making hydrolyzed plant protein results in MSG, so keep an eye out for the following in the ingredients statement:

- Autolyzed yeast extract
- Hydrolyzed plant protein
- Hydrolyzed soy protein
- Hydrolyzed vegetable protein
- Hydrolyzed yeast
- Protein isolate
- Soy extract
- Yeast extract

The FDA doesn't allow foods with these ingredients to have *No MSG* or *No added MSG* claims even if the source of MSG is natural. The FDA also states that MSG cannot be listed as *spices and flavoring*.

MSG is also sometimes called:

- Accent
- Ajinomoto
- Chinese seasoning
- Flavorings
- Gourmet powder
- Glutavene
- Glutacyl
- HPP
- HVP
- Kombu extract
- Mei-jing
- Monoammonium glutamate
- Monopotassium glutamate
- Natural flavoring
- RL-50
- Subu
- Vetsin
- Wei-jing
- Zest

Lactose (Sugar)

Lactose is a two-part sugar (aka a disaccharide) in milk, that is made of glucose and galactose. Lactose intolerance is a digestive intolerance to a sugar. For more on sensitivities to sugars, including other table sugar and fruit sugars, check out "Sugars" on page 66.

We don't know exactly how many people live with lactose intolerance, but some estimates indicate that 65 to 75 percent of people worldwide have some level of intolerance, with people of East Asian heritage being affected the most (50 to 100 percent) and those of Northern European descent being affected the least (5 to 15 percent). A 2010 consensus statement on lactose intolerance from the US National Institutes of Health (NIH) says that we don't know for sure how many people are affected. If you are not actually sensitive to lactose, you may be cutting out a food group with important nutrients; but if you do have a sensitivity to it, it's important to manage it, and there are plenty of alternative sources of the nutrients found in dairy foods.

Does human milk have lactose in it? Are babies ever lactose intolerant?

Human milk is about 6 percent lactose, which is a greater percentage of lactose than there is in cow's milk, which is about 4 percent lactose. Just about all babies have enough lactase enzyme to digest the lactose in breast milk. Very rarely, a baby is born without the enzyme. Most people naturally start to lose the ability to make lactase, starting from the weaning years into childhood and adolescence, though it varies by ethnicity. In fact, just about all ethnicities except for Northern Europeans have a large percentage of people with lactose intolerance. Lactase enzyme deficiency can start as early as age two, though symptoms of intolerance usually start to show up around ages six to ten. Secondary lactase deficiency can occur in adults, children, and even babies when the digestive tract is damaged by an infection, celiac disease, inflammatory bowel diseases, surgery, or sometimes medications (e.g., antibiotics). The cells that normally produce lactase are on the surface of the digestive tract, so when it is damaged, the body can easily become temporarily lactose intolerant. Once the digestive tract is healed, it should return to its previous level of lactase production.

> ## Lact- = Milk?
>
> When you see *lact-*, you ordinarily think "milk." However, *lact-* doesn't necessarily mean "lactose." And in fact, lactic acid, lactalbumin, and lactate are lactose-free. They may not be milk-free (lactic acid is milk-free, but lactic acid starter culture is not; milk allergy sufferers need to avoid lactalbumin; lactates are milk-free), but they are lactose-free. Casein is another word associated with milk, and it too is lactose-free (but contains milk proteins).

Lactose intolerance can be uncomfortable and painful for the sufferer. The most common symptoms are stomach pain, diarrhea, and gas, but symptoms can also include bloating, nausea, and vomiting. Unlike most food allergies, symptoms don't appear right away. It can be minutes or hours before symptoms appear, but it is most commonly reported that symptoms start thirty minutes to two hours after eating a trigger food. Strangely enough, yes. In certain cases, people can eat lactose without symptoms even when it fails to be digested or absorbed. That is, lactose intolerance is defined by the onset of symptoms. A person may lack enough lactase to digest lactose, yet not feel the classic symptoms such as abdominal pain, diarrhea, and gas. It seems this "lactose tolerance" is more common in people of European descent.

The level of lactose your body will tolerate depends on how much lactase it has available. Lactose intolerance is a dose-dependent condition: the more lactose over your individual limit that you consume, the greater your symptoms. When there is not enough lactase enzyme to digest lactose, the undigested lactose moves into the large intestine (aka the colon) and causes undesirable symptoms due to poor digestion and poor absorption of lactose. First, the concentration of lactose in the colon draws water from the body, flushing it into the colon to try to restore osmotic balance, but this results in diarrhea and therefore dehydration from all the water lost. The process to control osmotic balance is called osmoregulation, which is the body's way of keeping fluids from getting either too diluted or too concentrated. Second, lactose in the colon is food for the microbes that live there, and when microbes

> ## Lactose, Lactase: Which is Which?
>
> A quick tip for recognizing the names of sugars is that they often end in -ose. Lactose is a sugar. Enzymes, on the other hand, often end in -ase. Lactase is the enzyme that breaks down lactose.

consume lactose, the process creates gas and acids, which can lead to the body passing gas, accompanied by abdominal bloating and pain. The acids can also increase movement and water in the large intestine, which also contributes to diarrhea. Lactose intolerance is different from milk allergy.

If you're living with lactose intolerance, you probably know it. But sometimes the symptoms can mimic the symptoms of other conditions, such as inflammatory bowel syndrome, so it can be useful to get a proper diagnosis. Luckily, there are several options. A challenge could be done in a health care professional's office. Or you could have a test that is like a Breathalyzer except that it detects lactose. (Actually, it tests for hydrogen, which is a byproduct of undigested lactose. Any sugar that isn't digested will provide a positive result. But a test with a clinician in which lactose was the only thing eaten after a fast could improve the accuracy of the test.) Another choice would be a blood glucose test, which would show if lactose had broken down into glucose and galactose and the blood glucose had risen. A different test would be a biopsy of the small intestine to test for lactase activity; this is invasive, so your physician would rarely recommend this. Alternatively, a clinician could test your stool for undigested lactose. Finally, you could try an elimination diet. Any combination of these tests would give you a good idea whether you are sensitive to lactose.

The key to avoiding lactose is to know that only milk contains lactose. Any mammal milk qualifies. This includes human breast milk, cow's milk, goat's milk, and sheep's milk. Milk is made of casein (solids) and whey (liquids). Most of the lactose is in the liquid part of the milk (aka whey), though foods that are mostly casein, such as cheese, can still have some small amount of lactose. Soft cheeses, such as many goat cheeses, feta, mozzarella, and queso fresco, usually have more whey than other cheeses.

The good news is there are options for a lactose-free diet, from lactose-free versions of your favorite dairy foods to dairy alternatives. If you love milk and dairy foods, on top of this good news is the fact that many people can tolerate some lactose, so managing your condition is about keeping your overall lactose intake below your personal limit, not eliminating lactose. The 2010 NIH consensus statement found that 12 grams of lactose caused either no or minor symptoms in people with lactose intolerance (the amount in 1 cup of milk). It's easier to tolerate lactose if it's in a mixed food. Lactose-free milk is available and lactase tablets can be taken before eating. Many dairy foods don't have a lot of lactose in them because of the way they're made. For example, harder cheeses are virtually lactose-free (the sugar lactose is mostly in the watery whey, but cheese is made from the casein curds), and butter also has little lactose in it. For those looking for dairy alternatives, there are a number of plant-based milks, including almond milk, soy milk, and rice milk; there are also

> ### Sugars at a Glance
>
> disaccharide = di ("two")
> + saccharide ("sugar")
> = two sugars
>
> *sucrose*
> = glucose + fructose
>
> *lactose*
> = glucose + galactose
>
> *maltose*
> = glucose + glucose
>
> *monosaccharide*
> = mono ("one")
> + saccharide ("sugar")
> = one sugar
>
> *glucose*
> *fructose*
> *galactose*

yogurts, cheeses, and frozen desserts made from these plants. It's important to note that these may not be nutritional equivalents but that they are replacements for practical uses—when you want milk for cereal or coffee, or a cold dessert on a hot day, for example. A qualified health professional can guide you to make sure you are getting enough of the key nutrients found in dairy foods, such as calcium and protein.

To make sure you're getting enough calcium on a milk-free diet, find natural sources of calcium in edamame (young green soybeans), almonds; figs; bone-in fish, such as sardines or canned salmon with bones; soybeans; black-eyed peas; and some leafy greens, such as collard greens, turnip greens, kale, spinach, beet greens, and bok choy. Calcium-fortified foods include juices, soy milk, and tofu (prepared with calcium sulfate), rice milk, cereals, and breads. The daily recommended amount of calcium is 1,000–1,300 mg for most adults. The foods listed here typically contain at least 100 mg per serving, making them a good source of calcium; some foods listed are in the 300–400 mg per serving range (e.g., bone-in sardines, fortified orange juice, fortified soy milk, tofu made with calcium sulfate, fortified cereals can vary above and below this range check the label for specifics). Eating a variety of calcium-rich foods throughout the day can help meet daily needs.

Lactose Intolerances Versus Milk Allergies

Both will cause negative digestive issues, such as gas, stomach pains, diarrhea, nausea, vomiting, and bloating. A milk allergy may affect other systems in the body, the way any allergy might: runny nose, congestion, hives, and so on. In terms of what is going on inside the body, the milk allergy is an immune response to a protein in milk; lactose intolerance, on the other hand, is the body's reaction to poorly digesting and absorbing a sugar found in milk. It's possible for someone to have both a lactose intolerance and a milk allergy, and it's even possible for the immune reaction to a milk allergy to cause secondary lactase deficiency. A milk allergy is much harder to manage than lactose intolerance, so it's important to figure out which one is causing your symptoms.

Sugars

Table sugar, also known as sucrose, is probably the most familiar sugar. And yes, it is possible to have an intolerance—though not an allergy—to it. It is a disaccharide, which means it has two simpler sugars (monosaccharides), which are joined together (and need to be separated during digestion by specialized enzymes). Sucrose is made up of glucose and fructose. Other disaccharides that can be behind an intolerance are lactose (made up of glucose and galactose) and maltose (made up of two glucose molecules).

> ### Enzymes by Any Other Name
>
> You may encounter different names for the enzymes that break down disaccharide sugars. Remember that -ose is a sugar and -ase is an enzyme. Here are the pairs (the name of a sugar, followed by the name of the enzyme that breaks it down):
>
> - sucrose/sucrase
> - lactose/lactase
> - maltose/maltase
>
>   However, there are other names for the same enzymes. Here's a quick guide, just in case you encounter these other names.
>
> - Sucrase aka sucrose alpha-glucosidase
> - Lactase aka beta-galactosidase
> - Maltase aka alpha-dextrinase, glucoamylase, or isomaltase

Normally, disaccharides are split into their smaller components in the earlier phases of digestion in the small intestine, which is where the smaller components (monosaccharides) are easily absorbed. Under normal circumstances, the small intestine would be equipped with the right enzymes to break down each of the disaccharides, followed by normal digestion and absorption.

The sugar sucrose is broken down into glucose and fructose by the enzyme sucrase. For lactose, it is split into glucose and galactose by the enzyme lactase. The sugar maltose is broken down into two glucose molecules by the enzyme maltase. When the body does not have any, or enough, of the right enzyme to digest one of these sugars, the disaccharides move into the large intestine intact, resulting in symptoms such as gas, stomach pain and bloating, diarrhea, and sometimes even nausea and vomiting. It's also possible to have an intolerance to one of the monosaccharides, such as fructose.

See "Lactose (Sugar)" on page 63 for a discussion of lactose intolerance. Sucrose intolerance works in the same way lactose intolerance does. When there is not enough sucrase enzyme to digest sucrose, the undigested sucrose moves into the large intestine (aka the colon) and causes undesirable symptoms due to poor digestion and poor absorption of sucrose. First, the concentration of sucrose in the colon draws water from the body, flushing it into the colon to try to restore osomotic balance, but this results in diarrhea and therefore dehydration from all the water lost. Second, sucrose in the colon is food for the microbes that live there, and when microbes consume sucrose, the process creates gas and acids, which can lead to the body passing gas, accompanied by abdominal bloating and pain. The acids can also increase movement and water in the large intestine, which also contributes to diarrhea.

Sucrose is table sugar, which is often made from sugar beet or sugarcane. This means that many processed foods containing sugars will contain sucrose. Sucrose is also found naturally in many fruits, vegetables, and whole grains, from dates, mangoes, pineapple, oranges, and apples to corn, beets, peas, and carrots to rye, buckwheat, brown rice, and cornmeal.

Maltose is a sugar in starchy foods, including foods made with refined flours, such as white bread, pastas, flour tortillas, crackers, pancakes, and bagels. Starches are made up of larger compounds of many glucose molecules joined together, and these are broken down to the smaller maltose (two glucose molecules). During normal digestion, maltose is further broken down to two separate individual glucose molecules, and it's this "free" glucose that gets absorbed by the body. However, without enough of the enzyme maltase, the maltose will enter the large intestine (colon), where bacteria will consume it, creating the typical symptoms of sugar intolerance (gas, bloating, and diarrhea).

Fructose is a monosaccharide, or a simple sugar. Fructose intolerance works differently than disaccharide intolerance. Rather than an irregularity in the digestion (breakdown) phase of the process, fructose intolerance is usually the result of something going wrong in the absorption phase.

The exact mechanism is not completely understood, but it seems that under normal conditions, glucose helps the body absorb fructose. This means that when it comes to sucrose, in which glucose and fructose are present in equal parts, fructose is fully absorbed. However, when there is more fructose than glucose, any fructose not "matched" by glucose isn't absorbed and moves, intact, into the large intestine to create symptoms seen with other sugars that make it there. Interestingly, the body does not usually do a great job of absorbing fructose, and anyone who eats a lot of fructose will experience negative side effects: gas, abdominal bloating, pain, and diarrhea. There are a few well-known, though rare, inherited reasons for fructose intolerance, including a deficiency in an enzyme called fructose-1,6-bisphosphatase and a deficiency in an enzyme called fructokinase.

Fructose makes it into our diets in a few main forms. First, fructose can be consumed in its pure form as just fructose. In addition, it can be consumed as part of sucrose. As fructose makes up half of sucrose, any food with sucrose (glucose + fructose) in it will also contain fructose. Finally, fructose is sometimes part of more complex carbohydrates called oligosaccharides and polysaccharides; they're considered dietary fiber and aren't easily digested, and in fact are often used as prebiotics (food for good bacteria in the digestive tracts). Some foods contain more fructose than glucose; these include apples, pears, watermelon, honey, and high-fructose corn syrup.

FODMAP

In the realm of food intolerances, you may come across the acronym FODMAP, which stands for fermentable oligosaccharides, disaccharides, monosaccharides, and polyols (sugars and sugar alcohols that are fermentable; in other words, they are used as food by the bacteria in the gut). FODMAP describes a group of carbohydrate and sugar alcohols that the body has trouble absorbing and which are therefore left to be consumed by the gut bacteria, resulting in symptoms common in food intolerances (gas, abdominal bloating, stomach pain and cramps, and diarrhea). FODMAP foods don't represent food intolerances in the way we are discussing them in this book, because with enough of them, anyone would experience the negative symptoms. But sometimes a FODMAP diet—a diet that avoids large amounts of FODMAPs—is used with digestive conditions, such as irritable bowel syndrome (IBS), to manage symptoms.

Histamine and Tyramine

Though proponents of a Mediterranean diet would be sad to hear it, components of wine can cause negative reactions. It's not wine specifically that offends; it's substances that are commonly found in wine and other alcoholic beverages. These compounds are also often found in vinegars, fermented foods (such as pickles), some fruits, vegetables, spices, artificial colors, yeast extracts, and chicken liver. Histamine and tyramine are the culprits. The results include hives, itchiness, swelling, reddening, headaches, migraines, and stomach upset.

Histamine Intolerance

About 1 percent of the population has a histamine intolerance, and four out of five of them are middle-aged. Histamine intolerance is underdiagnosed, mostly because the symptoms are so similar to an allergic reaction that a physician might suspect allergies first and foremost. It is hard to diagnose because symptoms often show up hours after the histamine threshold has been reached, so an in-office food challenge won't show an immediate reaction, unless the patient is under observation for hours and is given increasing levels of histamine.

Histamine is a naturally occurring chemical that is biologically active, which means that it plays a role in many of the body's functions and is made by many of the body's cells. The chemical is also found in some foods. Histamine is involved in all inflammatory reactions, including allergic reactions. When histamine is released, it causes sneezing, itching, hives, and watery eyes. But histamine is also involved in the day-night sleep cycle, healing of wounds, and stimulation of gastric acid, to name a few of its roles. When the body is not able to break down histamine in foods quickly enough, histamine intolerance occurs. Symptoms of histamine intolerance are a lot like those of an allergic reaction; that's because histamine is involved in the allergic response. This may be why histamine intolerance is often misdiagnosed. Under normal circumstances, histamine is one of the body's first lines of defense. It lives in white blood cells and is the first thing that is released in response to inflammation. It helps the body fight bacteria and viruses by increasing blood flow and aiding the healing process. During this response, if the body is not able to break down histamine quickly enough, it builds up. When the level reaches a threshold point (which varies among individuals), symptoms start to appear. Under normal circumstances, histamine is easily broken down by two specific enzymes, and this takes place both in the blood and in the gut, so that we don't have to worry about the level of histamine in the foods we eat. With histamine intolerance, one or both of the enzymes can't break it down fast enough, causing symptoms.

The ability to convert histidine to histamine is fairly common among bacteria that exist in nature (e.g., in the gut of fish), so many natural foods contain histamine. For example, as soon as a fish dies, the tissue in its gut starts to break down, releasing histidine, which turns into histamine. That's the main reason it is important to gut a fish as soon as possible. Leaving it undone can mean excessive levels of histamine, which can double every 20 minutes. Shellfish don't get gutted, so it's more likely that they'd get to the plate with high levels of histamine if they're not processed correctly. This is one more reason to get to know your food providers and buy from reputable sources.

Fermented foods and drinks, including cheese, alcohol, vinegar, sauerkraut, soy sauce, pepperoni, bologna, salami, and frankfurters, contain histamine. For an unknown reason, some fruits tend to have more histamine when they are riper, including tomatoes, citrus fruits, berries, and tree fruits, such as stone fruits. And for some reason, riper eggplants and pumpkins tend to have more histamine. Cut or peeled fruits and vegetables tend to be higher in histamine because cutting them gives bacteria more access to the food. Egg whites and some food additives also tend to have more histamine than most substances.

Histamine is an important part of inflammatory reactions, so histamine is wherever inflammation is, including allergic reactions, infections, and even minor scrapes and bruises.

Somewhat confusingly, histamine intolerance feels a lot like a food allergy. The easiest way to differentiate the two is to think of food allergies as a more immediate concern, which can be triggered with even a small amount of the offending food. In other words, with a food allergy, a small amount of the allergen will set off the allergic reaction, leading to immediate symptoms. With histamine intolerance, the level of histamine has to build up to and past the threshold, so symptoms might not present themselves right away. In fact, sometimes it can take hours. These symptoms include itching, hives, swelling, a drop in blood pressure, a racing heart, panic attacks, chest pains, congestion and a runny nose, watery red eyes, headache, fatigue, confusion and irritability, heartburn, indigestion, and acid reflux. A histamine intolerance could worsen a preexisting condition, such as allergies, eczema, an allergy to something else entirely, inflammation, hormonal ups and downs of the menstrual cycle, or side effects from medications. Of course, not everyone has all of these symptoms, and some symptoms may be mild.

Similar to diagnosis for other food sensitivities, figuring out if you have a histamine intolerance starts with a good medical history, food and symptom tracker, and exam. A physician might help to rule out other causes of your symptoms. If you suspect a histamine intolerance, talk to your health care team, including a qualified registered dietitian, about it. They can put together a histamine-restricted elimination diet for you. The process is similar to the basic process outlined in this book; the differences will be in the specifics of what foods to include and exclude.

Following the elimination diet in this book carefully will help you identify some trigger foods, if not provide a diagnosis, and will give you good data to take to a registered dietitian, with whom you can plan the next steps.

Healthy people normally have 1 nanogram per milliliter (or less) of histamine circulating in the body. People with a histamine intolerance might start feeling symptoms in the 1ng/mL range, but it also depends on their personal threshold. Interestingly, everyone would experience some symptoms if they ate very large amounts of histamine-containing foods. An individual's histamine threshold can be lowered during infections, when experiencing hormonal changes during a menstrual cycle, and because of medications.

If I'm sensitive to histamine, do I have to avoid all foods that contain it or cause the body to release histamine?

Yes and no. Histamine intolerance is dose dependent. This means that the body has to reach a certain amount of total histamine before it reacts. It is only when the body has more than it can break down that symptoms show up. So management of a histamine intolerance will limit foods high in histamine, but they don't necessarily have to be completely cut out of the diet forever. However, because histamine doesn't come just from foods but also from inflammation and seasonal allergies, it can be challenging to predict the body's level of histamine at any given time. Your health care professional may recommend a histamine-restricted diet to try to keep your total histamine level under your threshold level.

Any food that uses microbial fermentation will probably have histamine, including cheeses; alcoholic beverages; vinegar; fermented vegetables, such as sauerkraut, kimchi, and pickles; fermented soy products, such as soy sauce; and processed meats, such as pepperoni, bologna, and salami. Histamine has also been found in citrus fruits, berries, tomatoes, stone fruits (apricots, cherries, and plums), and even some vegetables, such as eggplants and pumpkins. In general, the riper a fruit, the higher the level of histamine. We don't quite know why, but we also see histamine released in reaction to egg whites and some food additives, such as tartrazine (food dye), benzoates (preservatives), and sulfites (preservatives). It also occurs in reaction to seafood that hasn't been cleaned properly.

The following foods should be avoided on a histamine-restricted diet:

- Alcohol

- Certain food additives (tartrazine, artificial colors, benzoates and sulfites, all preservatives, and medications that contain any of these)

- Certain fruits (apricots, cherries, citrus fruits, cranberries, currants, dates, grapes, loganberries, pineapples, prunes, raisins, raspberries, and strawberries)

- Certain vegetables (avocados, eggplants, olives, pickles, pumpkin, spinach, tomatoes and tomato products, red beans, and soy and soy products)

- Chocolate

- Cocoa

- Cola

- Eggs

- Fermented foods (soy sauce, miso, vinegar, and sauerkraut)

- Fish

- Meat

- Milk and milk products

- Nonalcoholic versions of alcoholic beverages

- Some spices (chili powder, cinnamon, cloves, curry powder, nutmeg, and thyme)

- Tea

Barring outside fluctuations in histamine levels, such as seasonal allergies, controlling the amount in food and drink choices may help with long-term symptom management.

Tyramine Intolerance

Tyramine intolerance is uncommon except for those taking a class of antidepressant drugs called MAOIs (monoamine oxidase inhibitors). Monoamine oxidase enzymes regulate the amount of tyramine in the body, and MAOIs, as their name suggests, inhibit MAOs. Without the MAOs to regulate the amount of tyramine in the body, their levels could become quite high. When there is a lot of tyramine in the body, another chemical, called norepinephrine, also increases. It's actually the rise in norepinephrine that leads to symptoms, such as high blood pressure, rapid heartbeat, migraines, light-headedness, sweating, feeling hot, clamminess, chills, reddening, hives, and itchiness. Intolerance can occur without MAOIs being involved, but this is much less common.

Your health care team will work with you on specific recommendations for what to eat and not eat when taking an MAOI drug. There is debate in the field of health care about which foods to include and not include. Some lists are extensive and are considered overly restrictive. Here is a list of the foods that should be completely avoided:

- Aged and cured meats
- Aged and hard cheeses
- Beer from a tap
- Broad bean pods

- Poultry and fish
- Sauerkraut
- Soy sauce and other soy condiments

- Tofu
- Yeast extract products, such as marmite, Vegemite, and Bovril

If you consume red or white wine or bottled or canned beer (including the nonalcoholic type), do so in moderation.

We don't know as much about tyramine sensitivity when MAOIs are not involved. Nevertheless, if tyramine is identified as a trigger food, it's best to avoid high-tyramine foods (see previous list) as well as some fresh foods (e.g., avocado, bananas, eggplant, figs, and tomatoes). Tyramine is found in many protein foods and, like histamine, is found in foods that are fermented; it also occurs in spoiled food, as the microbes will readily convert tyrosine into tyramine.

Nitrates and Nitrites (Preservatives)

Nitrates are naturally existing nitrogen compounds found in all plants, including fruits, vegetables, and grains. Nitrates are also in the soil and water, so the amount of nitrates in a plant depends on where something was grown and the farming practices used to grow it. Nitrates are also found in fish and dairy.

Nitrites are formed from spoiled nitrates in plants but are not normally found in plants. Nitrates and nitrites are used as preservatives to protect against botulism. They are also used as a color and flavor enhancer in processed meats.

For people who are sensitive to nitrates and nitrates, even small amounts can cause flushing, abdominal pain, headaches, or hives. On a food label, you might see them in compounds with potassium and sodium. For example, you might see nitrates listed in the ingredients panel as potassium nitrate or sodium nitrate. Similarly, you may find nitrites on the label as potassium nitrite and sodium nitrite. All of these compounds are found in nature, with the exception of sodium nitrite.

Processed meats are a common food source of nitrates and nitrites. This includes popular foods, such as hot dogs, sausages, pepperoni, bacon, ham, salami, and other lunch meats. They are also found in smoked fish, meat pâtés, canned meats, and some cheeses (e.g., Gouda).

Each individual's threshold level is different. If nitrates and nitrates are suspected as trigger foods (a good guess if, for example, you have bacon each morning, a hot dog come noon, and sausage each night), you can avoid these foods for several weeks to see if symptoms clear up. If they do, the elimination period can be followed up with a food challenge to confirm that it was probably a nitrate- or nitrite-containing food that triggered symptoms.

CHAPTER 7

Other Common Conditions Linked with Food

In some cases, foods make an underlying condition worse. In the case of a condition such as celiac disease, it is understood that those with the condition must avoid gluten-containing foods. However, there are other conditions where the connection between food and condition is less clear (e.g., chronic fatigue syndrome). This chapter presents an overview of some key conditions in which food choice may play a role.

Celiac Disease

Celiac disease is a condition in which the body's immune system attacks itself after gluten-containing foods have been eaten. For people with celiac disease, eating gluten damages the small intestine, making it hard for the body to absorb nutrients from food. Sometimes even the smallest amount of gluten can cause symptoms; other times, the small intestine can experience major damage with no symptoms. Unlike classic food allergies, the antibodies are not the IgE type, but the immune system is still involved. There are a few other names for celiac disease, including celiac sprue, gluten-sensitive enteropathy, nontropical sprue, and gluten intolerance.

An inherited condition that runs in families, celiac disease can start during childhood or adulthood. It is estimated that about 2 million people in the United States may have celiac disease. A 2012 study of nearly 8,000 people concluded that 1 in 141 people in the United States have celiac disease, and four out of five of them (83 percent) are not aware they have it. It is more common within an immediate family, so if a mother, father, brother, sister, son, or daughter is diagnosed, other family members may want to be tested. It is also more common in people who have type 1 diabetes or Down syndrome.

There have been many more diagnoses of celiac disease since 2004, when an NIH Consensus Panel concluded that celiac disease was underdiagnosed and provided a report on the accuracy of testing for celiac disease, how many people have it (including those who are not aware that they have it), and key strategies to manage the condition. The report brought much-needed attention to celiac disease. This has encouraged the growth of support groups, improvements in recognizing and diagnosing the condition, and new gluten-free products, which are now available in mainstream markets (some of them providing a real service and some of them just gluten-free junk food, but options nonetheless).

What does celiac disease feel like?

Celiac disease can cause both immediate and long-term issues. Most commonly, there are immediate digestive symptoms after someone with celiac disease eats gluten-containing food. Symptoms include stomach pain, gas, bloating, indigestion, diarrhea, fatty stool that floats, and vomiting, as well as broad symptoms, such as feeling very tired, mood changes, and poor appetite. Longer-term effects can be a result of the body not being able to get the nutrition it needs over time, for example, anemia, weak or brittle bones, itchy skin rash, and even infertility. Interestingly, some people with celiac disease do not feel sick or have symptoms, though most do have one or more symptoms. Many of the symptoms, such as stomach pain, gas, and bloating, are common to many conditions, so having these symptoms doesn't necessarily mean that someone has celiac disease. If a person with celiac disease follows a gluten-free diet, symptoms tend to clear up.

The good news is that some of the immediate symptoms—such as the stomach pain, gas, and diarrhea—will start to get better in just a few days after eliminating wheat, barley, and rye. It may be a matter of months or even a couple of years before most of the small intestine is fully healed. Eating gluten-free has to be a lifelong way of eating to keep symptoms and long-term damage away.

We used to think that a protein in oats might be involved in celiac disease, but after more than a decade of research, we know that oats are fine for people with celiac disease. The concern is when there is cross-contamination with wheat, rye, or barley, which could happen in the field, during transportation, during storage, or during milling and processing if the grains share machinery. So although it might not be the oats themselves, someone who wants to keep even trace amounts of gluten out of his or her diet should look for oats that are labeled "gluten-free." Oats are a healthy food with heart health benefits; eating them can be an easy way to include more whole grains in the diet.

Celiac disease starts with exposure to gluten. The word *gluten* is a general term for the allergy-triggering proteins in wheat, barley, and rye. In wheat, including durum, semolina, spelt, Kamut (a brand of khorasan wheat), eikorn, and farro, the gluten proteins are alpha-gliadins. In barley, the gluten proteins are hordeins. In rye, the gluten proteins are secalins. (These proteins are different from the proteins in these grains that cause a more classic allergy [with IgE types of antibodies]). Once the alpha-gliadins, hordeins, or secalins are in the digestive tract, the immune system damages the intestinal tissues; this is the signature of celiac disease. In other words, it damages the intestinal cells whose job it is to help absorb nutrients from food, and it also weakens the protective gut lining, which makes it easier for the outside world to get directly into the bloodstream (this is called leaky gut).

Barring a specific allergy to the gluten-containing food you're eating, there are other conditions where gluten may play a role, but this is a controversial subject. According to a 2012 review paper on the topic, people without celiac disease or a wheat allergy sometimes had varying levels of improvement in their symptoms when they removed gluten from their diets. The conditions included an itchy skin rash with bumps or blisters (known as dermatitis herpetiformis) and a digestive disorder called irritable bowel syndrome (IBS). We need more high-quality research in this area to prove the benefits of a gluten-free diet for people without celiac disease.

What Is Gluten-Free? The FDA Has an Answer

Gluten-free products have captured headlines and grocery shelf space. With the growing category of foods labeled gluten-free, the FDA decided it was high time to develop official guidelines about what it means to be gluten-free. Standardizing the definition of gluten-free is meant to provide assurance to people looking for gluten-free foods, so in August 2013, the FDA announced that it had finalized its definition. Product makers have a year from the date of this announcement to come into compliance.

The FDA specifies that for a food to be labeled gluten-free, it must have less than 20 parts per million (ppm) of gluten, which is the lowest level that can be consistently detected using validated scientific measuring tools. Although some people will want assurance that there is zero gluten in foods, the truth is that most people with celiac disease can tolerate foods with this very, very small amount of gluten. The new FDA guidelines are in line with those of other countries and international food safety groups.

Diagnosing Celiac Disease

Diagnosis, which includes blood tests and taking tissue samples (biopsy), has gotten much more sophisticated in the past decade. The blood tests usually come first, but results can sometimes show false negative or false positive readings. That's why a blood test should be followed by a biopsy to help confirm the diagnosis. Also, though it seems counterintuitive, it's important to stick to a regular diet until diagnosis is complete. That's because going gluten-free for several weeks before testing means that signs of celiac disease won't show up on tests, and it's important to have a solid diagnosis.

Getting the Nutrients Found in Wheat, Barley, and Rye

Although there are a variety of vitamins and minerals in these grains, the hardest part about avoiding them may be the vigilance you must exercise, because these grains, especially wheat, are very common in the US diet. However, these grains are not unique in the nutrients they provide, and a well-rounded diet should provide all the nutrients the body needs. Thankfully, there are many alternatives, such as rice, wild rice, quinoa, potatoes, buckwheat, corn, and more.

Irritable Bowel Syndrome (IBS)

IBS is a way to describe a group of symptoms that someone with IBS will experience together. The good news is that there is no inflammation or changes to the tissues in the digestive tract, so it is not damaged, unlike conditions such as celiac disease, ulcerative colitis, or Crohn's disease. The bad news is that symptoms can be frequent and unpleasant. Also known as colitis, mucous colitis, spastic colon, nervous colon, and spastic bowel, IBS is not a disease but a way to think about a set of symptoms.

Most studies show that about 10 to 15 percent of the population has IBS, which is significant. Some estimates go as low as 3 percent, but others go as high as 20 percent. For every man who has IBS, two women are affected. It mostly affects people younger than forty-five. More than two out of three people with IBS work with a health care professional for diagnosis and treatment.

Health care professionals and researchers alike aren't sure what causes IBS, but they recognize that it exists. Researchers think that it could be some combination of physical and mental health issues. Although we don't know the exact roots of IBS, there are some theories:

- People with IBS may have food sensitivities, but not food allergies, that lead to their IBS symptoms. The most commonly reported trigger foods and drinks are carbohydrate-rich foods, spicy foods, fatty foods, coffee, and alcohol. One hypothesis is that IBS symptoms may be caused by the body's decreased ability to absorb sugars or bile acids, which help break down fats and get rid of wastes.

- The brain and the gut aren't communicating clearly. Normally, the nerve signals between the brain and the small and large intestines help regulate the intestines so that they function normally. When there is a disruption in the way the brain and gut can talk to each other, it's possible that changes in bowel habits, pain, or discomfort (symptoms of IBS) can appear.

- The large intestine isn't moving the way it should. If the large intestine doesn't move quickly enough, constipation is the result. On the other hand, if it moves too quickly, that can lead to diarrhea. It may also move in spurts, called spasms, or sudden strong muscle contractions, which are painful. These are all symptoms of IBS that may be triggered by stress or eating (or both).

- The brain may be especially sensitive to pain related to the gut. There is a theory that people with IBS have a lower pain threshold for the normal stretching of the bowel that happens because of gas or stool, which results in the IBS symptom of abdominal pain.

• There may be a link between psychological stress and physical symptoms in the gut. Though the link is unclear, people with IBS are more likely to also suffer from panic disorder, anxiety, depression, and post-traumatic stress disorder. In general, digestive disorders, such as IBS, are more common in those known to have gone through past physical or other abuse, which suggests that people who have been abused might be expressing emotional stress through physical symptoms.

• Bacterial infections in the stomach and intestines can lead to IBS in some people, though not others. Researchers aren't sure why this is true, but they project that some other underlying condition might play a role (e.g., psychological problems or preexisting abnormalities in the digestive tract lining).

• Too many or the wrong type of bacteria might be colonizing the small intestine. The human body is able to naturally and beneficially coexist with many bacteria, especially in the gut. However, when there is small intestinal bacterial overgrowth (SIBO), the bacteria can produce excess gas, diarrhea, and weight loss. Quite a bit of research would need to be done in this area to prove a link between SIBO and IBS.

• Female reproductive hormones may make symptoms worse during menstruation. Symptoms often flare up more frequently for young women with IBS at this time. In contrast, women who have gone through menopause have fewer symptoms.

• Genetics may play a role, though it's not clear. Some studies have found that IBS is more common when there are family members with digestive issues. It's not clear, though, whether it actually runs in families or if family members are simply exposed to the same things that lead to IBS or if they are hyperaware of digestive symptoms because someone in their family has had them.

Stomach pain that is related to irregular bowel movements is one of the most common symptoms. With IBS, stomach pain will start with irregular bowel movements or with stool that is irregular (looser and more watery or harder and lumpier than usual). The stomach pain usually gets better after the bowel movement. Other symptoms include diarrhea, constipation, bloating, incomplete bowel movements, and passing of mucus. Symptoms often start after eating.

Though it's not the only treatment, changing the diet can definitely help if food is a main trigger of your IBS symptoms. Food choices and portion sizes are very likely contributing in some part to IBS symptoms, so addressing dietary changes is often part of managing IBS. For example, large meals can cause cramping and diarrhea, so choosing smaller portions may help. Avoiding foods that are high in fat, dairy, alcohol, caffeine, or artificial sweeteners and avoiding gassy foods, such as beans and cabbage, may help.

The International Foundation for Functional Gastrointestinal Disorders suggests that four foods commonly cause symptoms: insoluble fiber (the type commonly found in grains), chocolate, coffee, and nuts.

As long as it doesn't cause too much pain, gradually increasing fiber intake to 20-35 grams per day can help with constipation in IBS. Increasing fiber doesn't improve symptoms for everyone with IBS, and causes more symptoms than not in others, so treatment really has to be individualized. Ultimately, the individual will want to keep a food and symptom tracker to find what foods work for him or her.

Diagnosing IBS

Generally, if you are experiencing symptoms at least three times a month for more than six months, it may be a good idea to talk to your doctor about IBS. He or she will take a complete medical history and exam. Your doctor should ask about family members with digestive disorders, as well as ask about anything in your recent past that might be contributing to the IBS, such as recent infections, stressful events, or even medications. This is usually enough to diagnose IBS, though you might be asked to go through some blood work to rule out other conditions.

IBS Versus IBD

The simplest way to explain it is that **IBS** is mechanical while **IBD** (inflammatory bowel disease) is inflammatory. IBS is caused by a colon whose muscles aren't contracting right. People with IBS don't have the inflamed digestive tract that people with IBD suffer from. For IBD, inflammation in the gut is its calling card.

Migraines

If you've ever known someone who suffered from migraines, you probably know how debilitating migraines can be. We don't yet know the causes of migraines, which makes them challenging to treat. Although health professionals think that many things can trigger a migraine—from anxiety to sensitivity to light and sound—diet seems to both trigger and treat migraine headaches. There are also medications and other suggested therapies, such as stress management, depending on what is right for the individual.

Migraine headaches are three times more common in women than men and affect more than 10 percent of people worldwide, including both children and adults. Also, migraines are very likely inherited; up to 90 percent of people who get migraine headaches have a family history of them. Migraines in women may be related to hormonal changes during their menstrual cycle. Current science suggests that migraines are linked to genetic mutations in the brain, though we don't have the full picture yet. This is a departure from years past, when scientists thought that migraines resulted from changes in the blood flow in the blood vessels in the head.

About one out of three people who get migraines has a kind of warning system prior to the onset of a migraine headache: he or she sees spots, lines, or flashing lights. These vision abnormalities are called an aura. Sometimes the warning system comes in the form of tingling in the arm or leg. The migraine itself is a painful headache with intense throbbing and pulsing in one area of the head (or sometimes even the whole head), and it can last anywhere from four hours to three days if left untreated. Sometimes migraines trigger nausea and vomiting, as well as sensitivity to light and sound.

Many things may trigger migraines, with certain foods and food additives being just one part of the puzzle. When it comes to foods, migraine triggers are individualized, so that one person's migraine may be triggered by red wine while another person may be fine with red wine but is sensitive to MSG. Here are some of the more commonly reported triggers of migraine headaches:

- Hormonal changes for women: before or during menstruation, during pregnancy, or during menopause. Hormonal birth control may help or may make things worse.

- Foods: milk, chocolate, aged cheeses, salty foods, processed foods; skipping meals or fasting.

- Food additives: aspartame, MSG.

- Drinks: alcohol, especially wine; coffee and other highly caffeinated beverages, including energy drinks.

- Stress: at work or at home.

- Overstimulation: bright lights, bright sun, loud sounds, strong scents, such as perfume or smoke.

- Poor sleep patterns: too much or too little; jet lag.

- Overexertion: intense physical activity.

- Weather: changes in pressure systems.

- Medications: oral contraceptives; vasodilators, which relax the blood vessels and are used to treat high blood pressure.

One study found that milk and chocolate were the two most common food triggers for a migraine. Other suspected food triggers are:

- Avocado
- Banana
- Chicken liver
- Dry pork and beef sausages
- Egg white
- Eggplant
- Fava beans
- Fermented beverages, such as wine, beer, lager, and ale
- Fermented cheeses
- Fermented sausages

- Fermented soy products, including soy sauce
- Fish and shellfish
- MSG
- Nitrates in pepperoni, hot dogs, and luncheon meats
- Peanut
- Pickled herring
- Salad dressings
- Sauerkraut
- Smoked and pickled fish
- Sour cream
- Spinach
- Strawberry and chocolate
- Tomato
- Vinegar and foods made with vinegar, such as mustard
- Wine
- Yeast extract

However, food is usually not the one and only cause of a migraine, even though changes to the diet may bring some relief.

It is also possible for your food allergy to also be triggering a migraine. If this is the case, other symptoms of an allergic reaction are probably present (hives, rash, stomachache, cough and congestion, and so on). Elimination and challenge of the foods that may be triggering a migraine are a good way to figure out what your personal trigger foods are.

Diagnosing a Migraine

There is no rock solid diagnostic test to figure out what foods are triggering your migraine headaches. As with determining other food sensitivities, it may be helpful to go through the elimination diet process, including using a food and symptom tracker and setting aside a period of eliminating suspected trigger foods, followed by a food challenge.

Chronic Fatigue Syndrome (CFS)

According to the Centers for Disease Control (CDC), chronic fatigue syndrome (CFS) is "a debilitating and complex disorder characterized by profound fatigue that is not improved by bed rest and that may be worsened by physical or mental activity." They use a three-point definition of chronic fatigue syndrome from 1994, which defines chronic fatigue syndrome as lasting more than six months, affecting quality of life, and having at least four of the eight classic symptoms.

1. Severe chronic fatigue has been going on for at least six months in a row, and there are no other causes of that fatigue, such as regular exertion or other medical conditions that have fatigue as a side effect.

2. The fatigue is getting in the way of daily life and work.

3. The patient is experiencing at least half of the following symptoms (four out of eight) at the same time:

- An overall feeling of illness, discomfort, and lack of well-being after exercise, which lasts more than 24 hours.

- Waking up tired. Sleep does not refresh or rejuvenate the patient.

- Short-term memory loss and inability to concentrate.

- Muscle pain.

- Joint pain that isn't caused or accompanied by swelling or redness.

- Headaches of a new type, pattern, or severity.

- Tender lymph nodes in the neck or armpits.

- A frequent or recurring sore throat.

CFS affects more than one million Americans, including both men and women, but for every man with CFS, there are four women. It is more common in adults in their forties and fifties but can happen at any age. It seems to affect all ethnic and racial groups of all income levels. There might be a genetic link, as sometimes members of the same family have CFS.

People with CFS are overwhelmingly fatigued. Sleep doesn't seem to help. Working out or strenuous mental exertion makes it worse. In addition to the calling card symptom of severe tiredness, people with CFS often feel muscle pain, find it difficult to concentrate or remember things, have difficulty sleeping, and feel extremely fatigued for more than 24 hours after exercise.

Other symptoms that people with CFS report but that aren't part of the definition are the following:

- Abdominal pain
- Alcohol intolerance
- Bloating
- Brain fog
- Chest pain
- Chronic cough
- Diarrhea
- Dizziness
- Dry eyes or mouth

- Earaches
- Irregular heartbeat
- Irritable bowel
- Jaw pain
- Morning stiffness
- Nausea
- Night sweats and chills
- Psychological problems (e.g., depression,

irritability, anxiety, or panic attacks)

- Sensitivity to light or blurred vision and eye pain

- Shortness of breath

- Skin sensations (e.g., tingling)

- Weight loss

People with CFS have varying levels of functionality, but the quality of life for most people with CFS is dampened, whether they are at school, at work, or at home with family. It tends to hit patients in cycles, with periods of active symptoms followed by periods of feeling more or less OK.

Scientists around the world have researched CFS but have not been able to find a cause for it. They think that it could have multiple causes and so have studied infections, immune disorders, stress, trauma, and toxins as possible contributing conditions. We don't have answers but following are some current working theories.

About one in ten people who had been infected with three viruses (Epstein-Barr, Ross River, and Coxiella burnetii) had CFS-like symptoms after infection, and those with more severe symptoms during infection were more likely to develop CFS symptoms later.

We have inconsistent data on how the immune system and allergies are involved in CFS. For example, because CFS symptoms are similar to the symptoms a person feels when the immune system is fighting off an infection, one hypothesis is that CFS is caused by stress or a viral infection that leads to chronic inflammation. However, although people with CFS sometimes have autoimmunity types of antibodies, the tissue damage, opportunistic infections, and increased risk of cancer seen in people with autoimmune disorders aren't there. Not all people with CFS have allergies, though most patients report food and drink intolerances (e.g., alcohol).

The central nervous system responds to physical and emotional stress by changing how much of certain hormones are released. Some CFS patients make less cortisol than healthy people, making them more susceptible to inflammation. Sometimes people with fibromyalgia show similar hormonal imbalances. The cortisol levels of people with CFS may be depressed compared with the cortisol levels of healthy people, but they are still within the normal range, meaning that cortisol levels cannot be used to diagnose CFS.

Some CFS patients experience very low blood pressure, light-headedness, and worsened fatigue after standing for long periods of time or when in warm places, such as hot showers. These symptoms could indicate other blood pressure–related conditions, especially if there is also visual dimming or slow response time to others talking, or if symptoms worsen after changing the body's position (e.g., going from lying down to standing up), eating, drinking a lot of water, not drinking enough water, or increased activity.

Managing CFS is complicated because there is no cure or medication for it. The condition is very individualized in each person who suffers from CFS, and so the treatment must be. The main goal of treating CFS is to help relieve the most debilitating symptoms, the ones that disrupt the individual's life. For example, if poor sleep is contributing to fatigue, establishing good sleep habits will be an important part of treatment. It could include setting a regular bed time; avoiding daytime naps; creating an extended wind-down routine; making sure the bedroom is used only for sleep or sex; avoiding caffeine, alcohol, and tobacco; making the room quiet, dark, and a comfortable temperature; and even trying light exercise earlier in the day (at least four hours before sleep). In another example, if deep muscular and joint pain is one of the most important symptoms for the person with CFS to address, then pain can be managed with over-the-counter pain-relieving medications and stretching, gentle massage, heat, acupuncture, or other relaxation techniques. A dedicated team of health care professionals can help design a program to relieve the symptoms that are most disruptive to the daily life of the patient.

Although there is no published evidence directly linking poor diet with CFS, a healthy, well-balanced diet is likely to be helpful for anyone with a chronic disease. In particular, it may help to avoid caffeine, alcohol, and nicotine, because they can disrupt sleep. In addition, it's possible that going through a well-managed elimination diet process (complete with challenge phase) could be part of revealing any underlying food sensitivities that might be contributing to symptoms of the CFS, even if they aren't the direct cause of the CFS.

Diagnosing CFS

Diagnosing CFS is difficult. Many people feel one or more of the symptoms related to CFS at some point. Who hasn't felt extremely fatigued or woken up unrested at some point in their lives? The common nature of some of the symptoms is one of the biggest challenges in being able to diagnose it. Also, there is no lab test or biomarker for CFS the way that high cholesterol is a telltale sign of heart disease, or the way blood tests and skin patch tests at least point in the direction of a possible allergy diagnosis. Further, the cycling of feeling ill and then well makes the illness hard to pin down, and when patients visit a doctor, there might not be anything obviously wrong. Last but not least, people with CFS can have different sets of symptoms, more or fewer symptoms than the next CFS patient, or milder or more severe symptoms. It's no wonder that CFS has a low diagnosis rate, which is why the CDC thinks that for every person who has been diagnosed, there are four people who have CFS and don't know it.

After taking a detailed medical history and conducting physical and mental health exams, the first thing your doctor should do is attempt to rule out other possible causes. Then if you've had at least six months in a row of severe fatigue and you meet the other conditions outlined in the definition of CFS, your physician should consider CFS as a possibility.

The Chronic Fatigue and Immune Dysfunction Syndrome (CFIDS) Association of America hosts a number of patient resources on its website, including support group information, at www.cfids.org/resources/support-groups.asp.

EoE

EoE is easier to remember (and to say) than eosinophilic esophagitis, and so we will refer to this allergic disorder as EoE. First, let's break it down. It is a rare condition that can affect an estimated 1 in 2,000 people. Both children and adults can get EoE, and it is most common in white males and may be more common in family members. People with EoE often have other allergic disorders (e.g., asthma, eczema, or food allergies).

Eosinophils are a type of white blood cell that help fight off infection but can also build up and cause inflammation. The esophagus is the tube running between the mouth and the stomach, and *esophagitis* refers to inflammation of the esophagus. Those white blood cells don't belong in the esophagus, and when they build up, they can damage the esophagus. Doctors believe this type of inflammation in the esophagus is caused by allergies, but they don't know exactly what is causing the allergic reaction in EoE.

People with EoE experience gastrointestinal symptoms after eating, including nausea, vomiting, and abdominal pain. There may also be heartburn-type symptoms. Sometimes there are more severe symptoms, including difficulty with solid foods, where swallowing is challenging and solid foods can get stuck in the esophagus. Symptoms are a little different in different age groups. Children tend to have ongoing stomach pain, trouble swallowing, or vomiting. In teens and adults, trouble swallowing is the most common symptom. In fact, the esophagus can become so narrow that food can't get to the stomach—this is a medical emergency.

Many theories about what causes EoE point to food allergies. Interestingly, EoE is not an allergy to a specific food, but any food allergies and intolerances may trigger it, possibly by increasing the amount of white blood cells. Asthma and pollen allergies may be related to EoE in much the same way. There is some evidence that reducing allergenic foods can help relieve symptoms and reduce the white blood cell count in the esophagus. Elimination diets can be used to see if symptoms lessen.

It's considered a lifelong condition, so there is no cure, and the main goal of treatment is to feel better by addressing the symptoms. An elimination diet may be able to help reduce symptoms. Skin and blood tests can help suggest possible trigger foods, but another tactic is to eliminate the eight major allergens (i.e., milk, eggs, wheat, peanuts, soy, tree nuts, fish, and shellfish). In extreme cases, a very restricted liquid diet might be prescribed. Although an elimination diet isn't easy, if it identifies the trigger foods, it can help in the long run because the patient will know what foods he or she can eat.

In a small study, 74 percent of the people who were on a diet that eliminated the eight major allergens had improved symptoms, and the inflammation in the esophagus went down, too. Another group in this study were fed a liquid diet (aka an elemental diet), and 88 percent of that group saw improvements. The elimination diet had an advantage in that it was able to offer real food without expensive supplements. For quality-of-life reasons, the elimination diet may be a better choice for some people, even though the elemental diet had slightly better results.

Diagnosing EoE

First, you'll want to rule out other reasons for eosinophils to be in your esophagus. Chronic acid reflux (aka GERD, gastroesophageal reflux disease), food allergies, and inflammatory bowel disease can lead to eosinophil white blood cells showing up in the esophagus. If other causes have been ruled out, the only way to test for EoE is by biopsy, in which a tissue sample from your esophagus is taken and analyzed. A physician will of course also take your medical history, and your history, along with the biopsy, will inform a diagnosis.

PART THREE
How to Do an Elimination Diet

CHAPTER 8

Preparing for an Elimination Diet

On a bare bones level, the elimination diet will include five phases: assess, plan, avoid, challenge, and change. The assessment phase includes keeping and analyzing a food and symptom tracker. The planning phase involves preparing yourself, your household, your kitchen, and your grocery lists for what you're about to do. The avoidance phase is when you are eating according to one of the plans in this book—the Targeted Elimination Diet or the Catchall Elimination Diet—and you are putting a lot of your preparation and planning into action. The challenge phase is when you start to reintroduce foods, one at a time, in to your diet to determine whether they are safe for you. The change phase is when you incorporate changes to the way you will eat for the long term, so that you can keep your symptoms at bay.

ASSESS: The process starts by keeping a food and symptom tracker. Record everything that passes your lips and any symptoms that develop. This is your baseline data. It should be an accurate reflection of your "before" diet, so eat the way you normally do.

ASSESS: Evaluate your food and symptom tracker. Look for patterns in the foods you eat, as well as in the types of symptoms you have. Identify what foods you eat the most often. Also, take note of what foods you eat before symptoms start to show up. If there are any clear links between foods and symptoms, make a note of these foods. During the elimination diet phase (the avoid phase), you'll ban them from your pantry. Keep in mind that sometimes symptoms take hours to show up and sometimes they are chronic (e.g., fatigue), and remember that it may not be possible to identify potential triggers right away. If your symptoms tend to fall into groups, make a note of that as well. For example, if your symptoms are stomach cramps, diarrhea, and bloating, make a note that you have digestive symptoms. Or if your symptoms are itchiness, hives, and rashes, then make a note that you have skin-related symptoms.

PLAN: Pick your path. At this point, decide if you want to try the Targeted Elimination Diet, adding on any strong suspects from your food and symptom tracker review. Alternatively, you may opt for the

Catchall Elimination Diet, which is more restrictive. This could be the right course if, for example, you have already tried the Targeted Elimination Diet but it didn't improve your symptoms.

PLAN: Prepare members of your household. The changes to your diet will affect the people in your home, so talk to them about what you're doing and why, and tell them how it will change the eating dynamics at home for a while. Talk about why you need to eat special meals that are different from everyone else's, why you'll have special foods in the pantry and refrigerator for the next few weeks, or why you need to eat at home and not at restaurants for the time being. If you cook for your household, it may mean cooking two meals or having someone else cook for the household, so that it's less likely that you'll breathe in any allergens through steam.

PLAN: Prepare yourself for the challenges. This book helps you with tip sheets (found in Chapters 15 and 16), but you must prepare yourself mentally. Read through the worksheets on common challenges and strategies for overcoming them. For example, know that sometimes symptoms flare up and seem worse at the start of an elimination diet before they improve. Acknowledge that there will be difficult times but that they will be temporary, and the end results will be worth it.

PLAN: Prepare your kitchen. If it's possible, clear out all the trigger foods in the house. For nonperishable items, perhaps store them out of sight until the challenge phase. If that's not acceptable to other people in your household, try to create a separate space for your elimination diet foods, and assure everyone that it is temporary.

PLAN: Prepare your menus and your grocery lists. This part is done for you! To make a challenging process a little easier, use my menu plans, recipes, and grocery lists to guide you through your elimination diet. The only adaptations you'll have to make is if the menu includes a food you've identified in your food and symptom tracker evaluation.

AVOID: Eliminate and track. It's important to go through all the preparation steps rather than jump right into the elimination diet. You're more likely to succeed if you have a plan and are ready to face the ups and downs of an elimination diet. Now that you are ready, work your way through the menu plans, and be sure to track your symptoms and whether they are showing up more often or less, if they are getting more severe or improving. Also, track how you are feeling overall: tired, energized, achy, and so on. You can use the worksheets provided in this book. The Targeted Elimination Diet takes four weeks. The Catchall Elimination Diet takes two.

AVOID: Have your symptoms improved? If the answer is yes, proceed to the next step. If the answer is no, it's time to look at your food and symptom tracker and eliminate more foods, starting with your most commonly eaten foods. Try this for one week. If your symptoms have improved, move to the next step; if not, repeat the process by cutting out more foods. If this still does not clear up your symptoms, you may consider that food is not behind your symptoms after all.

CHALLENGE: Challenge and track. After the elimination diet period, it's time for the challenge and track phase. It is important to keep up with your food and symptom tracker at this time because this is when you will get the best picture of what foods are causing your symptoms. It's also important to add back one food at a time into your diet. For the food challenge, you will be eating a small amount of the potential trigger food in the morning and then monitor for symptoms. If there are no symptoms, you will increase the amount you eat at lunch and again monitor for symptoms. If again there are no symptoms, you will increase the amount of the food even more and eat it at dinner. For the next three days, you will go back to the original elimination diet, monitoring for any delayed symptoms. You can add this food to your "safe" list, but don't include it in your diet until all the food challenges are done. If symptoms did develop, go back to the elimination diet until symptoms improve before testing the next food. Repeat for each challenge food.

CHANGE: Create your maintenance diet. Use your elimination diet as the foundation for your maintenance diet, adding the foods that you've newly discovered as "safe" and eliminating for the long term any foods you discovered contribute to your symptoms.

A few additional considerations:

- Think about seeing a specialist (e.g., a gastroenterologist or an allergist) to confirm any food allergies or intolerances.

- You might want to make an appointment with a registered dietitian to make sure you are getting all the nutrients you need on your maintenance diet.

- You may wish to test trigger foods every once in a while. Some allergies and intolerances aren't necessarily forever. It's possible to reintroduce a trigger food back into the diet at some level after you've let the body heal for six months. Consider repeating challenges at that time.

Assess: Start Your Food and Symptom Tracker

Get ready: You are about to become intimately familiar with everything that you eat.

It's tempting to think of the initial food and symptom tracker as something that is done before you get started on the elimination diet, but the truth is that the baseline observation phase is just as important as any other step in the elimination diet and is integral to your overall success. You should treat it with the same attention and dedication that you'll give to the rest of the program. Ideally, record at least a week of data. If you are able to do it, track two weeks of data. There are worksheets in Chapters 13 and 14, but any way that works for recording your eating habits and the effect food has on you is fine.

You do this so that you can know, with as much accuracy as possible, whether what you're doing is making a difference. You record what you eat, when you eat it, and how it makes you feel. Be aware that the act of observation tends to change what is being watched. This is known in the world of physics as the observer effect. Keep in mind that this baseline observation phase is not the time to change. This is the time to be very much in tune with your body. It's not the time to make drastic changes in what you eat.

How to Keep Your Food Journal

If you've ever kept a food journal, this will look familiar. But because the food journal is a vital part of the elimination diet, it is more accurately described as a food and symptom tracker. That said, if you haven't kept a food journal before, you'll be a pro by the time you've completed your elimination diet.

I cannot say this too often: Keeping a food journal may be tough at times, but it is essential to the elimination diet. This is why I'm going to walk you through the basics of keeping a food journal. Be sure to read through all the instructions before you start, and come back to them if you ever need a refresher. It's important to do this part right. That said, it's fairly straightforward. Substitute "foods" for "boys" or "girls," and it's like a teenager's journal in that you will be taking careful notes on what foods do and don't like you back.

The first time you keep a food and symptom tracker will be in the assessment phase, before you start the elimination diet. Keep your diet as close to your regular routine as possible. The idea is to record your typical diet, so we can see what veering away from it in the following weeks will do to how you feel. See the Sample Food and Symptom Tracker on page 145 for an example of what yours might look like.

Every time you eat or drink something, be sure you're answering these five questions:

1. What is it?
2. What's in it?
3. How much did I eat?
4. How do I feel?
5. Is there anything else going on?

What is it?

Write down everything you swallow, whether it's food, drink, supplements, or medication. Do it in real time. Don't wait too long or you may forget important details and could miss out on identifying your personal trigger foods. You'll also want to jot down the time.

What's in it?

If you're eating something more complicated than, say, a banana, you'll want to break it down into its most basic ingredients, so that you'll have a better chance of figuring out your trigger foods. For example, for spaghetti and meatballs, you might record this: white pasta; store-bought marinara sauce with tomatoes, bell peppers, mushrooms, onions, carrots, salt, and pepper; fresh basil; meatballs made with ground beef, bread crumbs, egg, salt, pepper, and onion.

How much did I eat?

It's fine to use kitchen utensils to measure how much of a food you ate. For example, you could list the foods you ate in cups, ounces, tablespoons, pinches, and so on. It's important that you're comfortable with how you're measuring how much of a food you eat. Later, this will come into play as you figure out your personal threshold for a food, or how much of a food will trigger your symptoms.

If you had a yogurt parfait with granola and blueberries, you'll want to write down how much yogurt, how much granola, and how much blueberries you ate. There are also plates, bowls, glasses, and so on, with built-in measuring lines that I think are pretty clever but certainly not required. You can get them from elegantportions.com (simple, clear glass with etched lines), measureupbowl.com (basic white ceramic bowl with indented measuring lines along the inside), and preciseportions.com (uses vine graphics, if you're into that kind of thing).

How do I feel?

Check in with yourself after you've finished eating, and note how you feel. If you notice any symptoms developing, write them down immediately, and rate your symptoms on a scale of 1 to 5, with 5 being severe and 1 being mild. Be sure to jot down the time your symptoms start. Keep track of your symptoms, and also note down what time they start to fade away or are gone. Tips on how to describe your symptoms ("How should I talk about my symptoms?") follow.

Is anything else going on?

Make a note of anything else that's going on in your life or environment that you think could be affecting how your body reacts, whether it's stress; premenstrual syndrome (PMS); being around animals, gardens, or moldy places; having a cold; or even enjoying a hard workout.

Describing Symptoms

Following is a list of symptoms that people have reported in connection with food intolerances and allergies. If you have a symptom that is not on the list, write it down and keep track of it throughout the elimination diet. As long as you understand your own words and severity scale to describe your symptoms, you will be fine. The list that follows discusses common symptoms and may help you describe your symptoms. Take stock of your symptoms and rate them on a scale of 1 to 5, with 1 being mild and 5 being severe. You'll track your symptoms throughout this journey and come back to these baseline values to see what kind of progress you've made.

Skin

- Eczema (persistent dry and itchy rash)
- Hives (reddish, swollen, and itchy areas)
- Itchiness
- Numbness
- Rash
- Redness or flushing
- Swelling
- Tingling

Ears and Mouth

- Blurred vision
- Itchy ear canal
- Itchy mouth
- Odd taste in mouth
- Swelling of lips or tongue*

Digestive

- Bloating
- Cramps
- Diarrhea
- Gas
- Heartburn
- Nausea
- Stomach pain
- Vomiting

Nose and Head

- Congestion
- Headache
- Migraine headache
- Runny nose

Throat, Chest, and Lungs (Respiratory)

- Asthma
- Chest pain*
- Difficulty breathing
- Shortness of breath or wheezing*
- Slight, dry cough
- Sneezing
- Swelling of throat*
- Throat tightness
- Trouble swallowing*

Psychological

- Irritability
- Nervousness
- Sense of impending doom*

Other

- Dizziness
- Loss of sense of balance
- Turning blue*

- Drop in blood pressure (feeling faint, confused, weak, or passing out)*
- Loss of consciousness*
- Weakened pulse*

These symptoms are more severe, and if you are experiencing any of these, seek medical attention.

Nonconventional Descriptions of Symptoms

Describing your symptoms the way it makes sense for you is just fine. Following are some descriptions of how food sensitivities feel that may resonate for you. If so, feel free to describe your symptoms in this way. Or describe your symptoms in your own words.

- My lips feel tight.
- My tongue feels heavy.
- My tongue (or mouth) is tingling (or burning).
- Something feels like it's stuck in my throat.
- I just feel uneasy.
- My stomach always hurts.

- It feels like I have tiny cuts all over my lips.
- I've been having a hard time breathing.
- I feel mucous-y.
- Exercise makes me cough.
- I feel like I have to clear my throat all the time.
- My chest and back hurt.

Evaluating Your Food and Symptom Tracker

After you have accumulated at least a week's worth of data, it's time to evaluate your food and symptom tracker. No doubt you have been doing this informally along the way, but now is the time to take a look at the whole picture. It may be helpful to have a few different color pens or markers for this. First, take a look at the symptoms you've recorded, and pick the one that was consistently the most severe or painful. Next, see if you can identify anything similar about the foods that you ate prior to the symptoms. For example, let's say your food and symptom tracker shows that you have painful stomach cramps with bloating and then diarrhea three times over the week, and your meals prior to these incidents were milk and cereal on one day, chicken fingers and mozzarella sticks on another day, and tomato bisque soup on the third day. They all have dairy in common. In particular, they all have dairy that is heavier in lactose. In this case, dairy will already be eliminated from both the Targeted and Catchall Elimination Diets. However, when you go through the challenge phase, you can test with lactose-free or low-lactose dairy foods, such as lactose-free milk or a hard cheese, to see if your symptoms are dairy-related or just lactose-related.

If you'd like, you may repeat this for the second most severe symptom, and so on, to see what patterns emerge. However, be cautious with self-diagnosis in this phase, as you are about to eliminate many foods from your diet.

If your tracker identifies a potential trigger food for you that is also on the allowed foods list, you can personalize your diet by removing this food. The good news is that it is more likely that you are sensitive to just one or two types of foods than allergic to ten.

Pick Your Path

It's time to decide which of the two elimination diets you will try. To help you decide, take a look at the menu plans for the Targeted Elimination Diet (i.e., the one that includes more foods). This is probably the easier diet to follow, and it is the recommended diet unless you have noticed negative reactions clearly linked to many of the foods on the allowed list. If you notice more than five foods you react strongly to, you may want to try the Catchall Elimination Diet. The number five is somewhat arbitrary; you can decide what is best for you. Here are some pros and cons and also more information on types of eliminations diets:

TARGETED ELIMINATION DIET
Pros: With proper planning, this can be a nutritionally adequate diet for the long term.
Cons: Including more foods means there is a greater chance that you'll continue to be exposed to a food sensitivity, and it may take longer to identify this trigger food.

CATCHALL ELIMINATION DIET
Pros: It's useful when there it's not clear how food and symptoms are related.
Cons: It's very restrictive.

Although there are many variations of elimination diets, when it comes to the details of what foods are included and what foods are excluded, we will think of them in two categories: targeted and catchall.

What are Targeted Elimination Diets?
A Targeted Elimination Diet will eliminate targeted foods that have been identified as possible trouble foods. These diets could eliminate just one food type (e.g., dairy) or a select handful of food types (e.g., eight major allergens). Even diets that are more restrictive and eliminate additives, preservatives, or foods high in certain biologically active chemicals (e.g., histamine) are considered Targeted Elimination Diets.

These diets eliminate specific foods that are highly suspect for one reason or another, such as they have been singled out as possible culprits in the pre–diet phase food and symptom tracker, they are highly allergenic—perhaps one of the eight major allergens, or they have chemicals that have been identified as possible triggers, such as sulfites, benzoates, histamines, and so on.

Another common version of a Targeted Elimination Diet eliminates one major food type (e.g., dairy). This type of elimination diet is less restrictive than the two that will be outlined in this book. This means that if you decide you want to try eliminating only one (or two, or three, but not all eight) of the major allergens, you will have the tools you need to know how to read food labels, safely avoid the food, and find alternatives by using the targeted tip sheets in Chapters 15 and 16.

The single-food elimination diet is not really a true elimination diet, in the classic clinical sense. It is significantly simpler and is useful when you have a strong suspicion that a particular food may be the offending food. It is relatively easy to plan and follow, and it may be a way to dip your toe in the elimination diet waters. On the other hand, if your symptoms do not clear up, it's not much of a diagnostic tool. This diet is best used when you have a fairly strong idea of what the culprit is and you are looking for confirmation. To assess if this food is indeed your offending food, it should be part of your regular diet. During the seven days prior to the single-food elimination diet, keep a food and symptom tracker as you did with the other elimination diets, being sure to track when and what you eat and drink, and when and what symptoms you notice.

What are Catchall Elimination Diets?

Catchall Elimination Diets eliminate far more foods than Targeted Elimination Diets. The aim is to remove foods with the most allergenic or intolerance potential, so the remaining list of foods that are allowed is short.

These diets eliminate most foods and are useful when it's not clear what the trigger foods might be. To be effective, they must be very restrictive. They may not be nutritionally adequate for the long term, so it's important to think of the Catchall Elimination Diet as a short-term tool to identify trigger foods. If symptoms improve, the very least this diet can do is identify a handful of safe foods, which in itself is sometimes a huge relief.

The Catchall Elimination Diet takes two weeks. It's shorter than the Targeted Elimination Diet because it's hard to get all the nutrition you need. However, on a short-term basis, it is acceptable, especially if it helps set you up for long-term healthy eating.

Why would someone choose the Catchall Elimination Diet?

When you don't know what ails you, this type of diet can be helpful. A Catchall Elimination Diet includes only foods that tend to be safe for most people, though there is always a chance you will react to one of the foods on the allowed list. If this occurs, listen to your body and eliminate the trigger food.

Elemental Diets

If neither of these diets brings you any relief but you still think food is behind your symptoms, there is an option to eliminate all foods and drinks from your diet, replacing them with an elemental diet. The elemental diet is a short-term liquid diet that has predigested nutrients, particularly proteins that have been broken all the way down to amino acids. This diet provides all the essential macronutrients (carbohydrates, proteins, and fats) and micronutrients (vitamins and minerals) the body needs. During this time, the liquid formula is your only food, and all the solid food and even beverages normally consumed are taken out of the diet. These formulations usually don't taste great. There are a lot of reasons to try other options unless the elemental diet is the only medically advised option. Usually, elemental diets are prescribed by a health care professional and are not attempted without medical supervision. It's best to work directly with a registered dietitian or other qualified health care professional to make sure you are meeting all your nutrient needs.

CHAPTER 9

Plan and Eliminate

How well you can do anything depends on how well you are prepared for it. The secret to doing anything is to be ready for it, both mentally and physically. When you are about to dedicate hours to training for a race, rehearsing for a show, or studying for a test, you know that you are giving up other activities, that you need to find the energy to thrive in those hours, that you need the people in your everyday life to understand what you're spending your time and energy on, and that you need them to respect your commitment and support your decision.

Talking to the People in Your Household

It's important to share your plans to go on an elimination diet with the people you live with, because they will more than likely be affected, especially if you have any food buying or cooking responsibilities for the house. Here is a checklist of the topics it is useful to cover with members of your household. Depending on how comfortable you are about it, you may share more or fewer details about your symptoms; that is up to you. Basically, you will want to share why you're doing what you're doing, and then tell them how it might affect them.

- Tell them why you are going on an elimination diet. Maybe tell them about your symptoms, that you are looking for relief, and that you want to see if an elimination diet can help you identify foods that are contributing to the problem.

- Give them a list of foods you'll be avoiding and where they show up in prepared foods and beverages.

- Let them know how long it will last. Assure them that the most restrictive part of the diet is temporary and that your goal is health, not restriction. You simply want to feel better.

- Let them know that it's not going to be easy for you to make so many changes and that you realize it may be a burden on them at times, too. For example, they may suddenly need to cook separate meals, they may need to buy separate groceries, or they may be upset that you can't go out to eat with them for the time being. Tell them you're sorry for that but that it's temporary, that it's important to you to stick to this diet, and that you hope they'll be supportive.

• Share with them some of the changes regarding food and the kitchen that you're going to make, and emphasize that you need them to be OK with these changes. Some of the changes might be the following:

  • You will set up your kitchen so that you have your own cutting boards, meal preparation utensils, cookware, dinnerware, and silverware. You will also set aside a designated place to store these things, as well as a separate area to prepare your foods if possible.

  • You will dedicate a separate area of the pantry to the foods you can eat.

  • You will avoid cross-contact between your foods and others' foods. (Read more about cross-contact and how to manage it in Chapter 15).

  • You will prepare the elimination diet meal before the other meals.

Preparing Yourself Mentally

If you're thoroughly fed up with your symptoms and ready to go to great lengths to feel better, you may not need to do the mental preparation exercise to ready yourself for the challenges ahead. For most, however, it's a good idea. It's no fun being surprised with challenging situations. By going into the process with your eyes wide open, you may be better equipped to cope with it.

• Remind yourself why you are going through the elimination diet process. You might even want to write down your reasons. On that same sheet of paper, you could write down all the things you're willing to do to achieve your goal. (There's a handy Self-Efficacy Worksheet on page 120 for this.)

• Know that the symptoms you are working so hard to fix may actually worsen in the first two to four days. This is usually temporary and will pass. If it doesn't, you may want to talk to your health care team.

• Keep in mind that the elimination diet is not a cure-all. If food is related to your symptoms, the elimination diet may help identify those foods so that you can remove them from your diet and feel better. However, if your symptoms are not diet-related, the elimination diet won't help, and you should be ready to realize that. For example, if you haven't experienced any improvement in your symptoms in two weeks, you may want to put the elimination diet aside.

- Be aware that you should expect symptoms to improve but that they may not disappear entirely. Don't quit the process just because your symptoms don't vanish!

- Know that there are complex reasons why your elimination diet might not work, even if you truly do have a food sensitivity. Be aware of this potential outcome so that you can prevent it. For example, if the food you eat on the elimination diet comes into cross-contact with a food you have a sensitivity to, then you are not truly on an elimination diet and might not see improvement in your symptoms. Or you might have foods in your elimination diet that you are sensitive to. Although this is unlikely, especially if you're on the Catchall Elimination Diet, it is still remotely possible.

Get Your Kitchen Items in Order

Now that you are mentally prepared and have shared your plans with the other members of your household, it's time to get to work making some changes in your food environment, starting with the kitchen.

You will want to set aside your food and anything that touches it. It is very likely that life will not always be this way, but at this point, you may not know your level of sensitivity to a food, so it's best to be abundantly cautious during the elimination diet. Eventually, getting to know your personal limits with certain foods will be liberating. Instead of guessing, you will know how much of something you can have, and then you will be in control of keeping symptoms at bay.

Dedicate a portion of the refrigerator to your perishables. Perhaps you can claim a crisper drawer and a shelf. In general, the higher shelves are safer. Lower shelves may come into cross-contact with food that drops from higher shelves. (This is actually the reason that all people are advised to store raw meat on the lower shelves of a refrigerator.)

For your pantry staples, seek out a dedicated space in the pantry or perhaps a separate cabinet drawer. Again, if shelving is involved, the higher shelves will be safer for your food.

Select your cutting boards, knives, mixing spoons, food thermometer, pots, pans, and a place setting's worth of materials: plate, bowl, set of silverware, drinking glass, mug, and so on. It may be easier on you and your family if you have a separate set of anything that touches your food, because these items need to be cleaned carefully between uses. However, if you decide not to have separate pots, pans, dishes, and so on, be sure to thoroughly clean shared items with soap and water before using them in your food preparation.

Though nickel is not expressly limited in either elimination diet in this book, if you'd like to cut down on nickel exposure, use pots, pans, and containers made of iron, aluminum, or glass for food preparation and cooking. Avoid stainless steel and nonstick pots, pans, and containers; reactive chemicals can transfer from them to foods being cooked in them.

There is a checklist in the tools section (Chapter 12) of the more common kitchen items you may want to keep separate. The specific foods that will go into the refrigerator and pantry will depend on which elimination diet path you choose. Food lists are available in the Prep Your Pantry discussions in Chapters 13 and 14 for each elimination diet.

Eliminate and Track

Simply put, you are avoiding many foods, eating only specific foods, and recording it all along the way. The elimination period of the process can be explained simply, but it is a complex thing to live day to day. That's why this section includes some strategies for dealing with common challenges of the elimination diet.

As for what to eat, chances are that you have enough to think about during the elimination phase of the process. Leave the meal planning to me. You can use the meal plans and grocery lists that I've developed for the first weeks of each of the elimination diets. Of course, if you are feeling up to the task of developing meal plans, go ahead and jump to Chapter 17: Maintenance Diet Tools.

Is there a better time to start the elimination diet?

These are a few common questions people have about the elimination phase: Start when you'll have some time to yourself. Starting during holidays and celebrations may make a challenging process even more challenging. The first several days may bring harsher symptoms before they subside. Symptoms should start to clear by the end of the first week.

How do I cope with avoiding the foods I usually eat?

Pick substitutions from a similar category. For example, instead of milk, go for rice milk or oat milk. In chapter 15, there are suggestions for alternative foods according to use (e.g., rice milk instead of cow's milk), as well as according to key nutrients.

Will I be able to eat out at restaurants?

It's easier if you prepare your own foods, which you can bring with you. If that is not socially acceptable, you should be ready to educate the restaurant staff about your dietary restrictions. They may or may not be amenable to or capable of meeting your needs. Some restaurants tout the fact that they are sensitive to dietary restrictions. Call ahead and do some research on restaurants before venturing out.

How do I handle special occasions, such as birthdays and holidays?

It's a good idea to get in touch with the host in advance. It's respectful to simply explain your situation and ask about what will be served, assuring the host that you are more than happy to bring a dish that everyone (including you) can enjoy. Be aware that you may need to be vigilant about cross-contact.

Do I need to read food labels for foods I've already reviewed and figured out are safe for me?

Yes, you should hone your label-reading skills, and you should read labels every time you buy a food because ingredients could change without warning.

How do allergens get into my food without my knowing it?

• The same utensils are used to touch an allergen and your food or plate.

• Allergenic foods and nonallergenic foods are both processed on the same machinery, and the cleaning in between is inadequate.

• Labels can be misleading: A nondairy creamer often contains sodium caseinate.

• Ingredients are listed by their function rather than what's in them, such as emulsifier instead of egg white.

• An ingredient is listed but what it's made of is not specified, such as mayonnaise instead of olive oil, egg, vinegar, and salt.

• The manufacturer runs out of one ingredient, such as canola oil, so soy or peanut oil is used instead.

• There is such a small amount of the ingredient that it does not have to be listed on the label.

CHAPTER 10

Challenge Phase

Now that you've wiped the slate clean, it's time to reintroduce foods, one at a time, in order to figure out what ails you. You have to challenge your body with precise amounts of each food. Monitor for symptoms very carefully, and look for immediate reactions, which can be defined as within four hours. Delayed reactions will show up one to four days out.

Identifying Challenge Foods

For the Targeted Elimination Diet, you will be using foods from each of the food groups that have been eliminated as your challenge foods: milk (dairy), eggs, wheat, peanuts, soy, tree nuts, fish, and shellfish. You will also be using foods high in sulfites, benzoates, artificial colors, MSG, and lactose. Test foods have been identified for you in Chapter 13.

For the Catchall Elimination Diet, you will using the most commonly eaten foods from your regular diet first. There are worksheets in Chapter 14 to help identify your challenge foods.

What are the different ways to do a food challenge?

There are three basic approaches, but you will most likely be doing the third. The first two are done in a health care professional's office, and the third can be done at home.

1. Double-blind placebo-controlled food challenge: Usually, this is what is done in research studies and special clinics. Neither the patient nor the supervisor knows what is in the test food, and each test is compared with the patient's reaction to a placebo (usually a glucose powder) in a gelatin capsule similar to that of the food.

2. Single-blind food challenge: This is supervised by a physician, dietitian, or nurse in an office setting; the patient doesn't know what the food is, but the supervisor knows. The food is disguised in another, stronger-tasting food.

3. Open food challenge: This is the one you are most likely doing and so is the one I will give you the most guidance on. Just know that you have resources on your health care team should you need additional support. This is the challenge most commonly done at home. You need to know the amount and what you are eating. Do this only with foods you've eaten in the past without severe reactions or with foods that are unlikely to cause an anaphylactic reaction.

How to Do an Open Food Challenge

First, please note that an unsupervised open food challenge is not appropriate for anyone who has ever had an anaphylactic reaction. Many of the symptoms caused by food sensitivities, although uncomfortable, are not severe, which makes an at-home open challenge OK for most people. The concept is that you will be reintroducing a food rather than challenging with completely new foods. So it is safe to assume that these foods, even if they cause bad reactions, won't cause dangerously severe reactions. It's not a bad idea to have a health care professional supervise the process. A food challenge can take the better part of a day, so make sure you set aside enough time.

The process involves starting with a small amount of the challenge food, waiting and watching for symptoms, and then repeating the process with a greater amount of the food until either symptoms appear or you've doubled a regular serving. Worksheets are available in the Chapters 13 and 14 for each elimination diet to make the process simple and organized.

Other than the challenge food, you should stay on an elimination diet during and between all the food challenges. Once challenge foods are determined to be safe, add them to a list of safe foods, but keep them out of your diet until all the food challenges are done. Do this is to keep the results clean.

If symptoms (e.g., swelling, reddening, irritation, rash, runny nose, watering eyes, and so on) develop, it's time to stop the food challenge and record how much of the offending food you had eaten when symptoms started. Then go back to your elimination diet until the symptoms go away completely. After that, wait another forty-eight hours before doing another food challenge. This gives the body time to get rid of all the food that could cause a reaction.

However, if the challenge was completed without any symptoms appearing, simply watch for any delayed symptoms to appear by day two, at which point you are back on the elimination diet and the challenge food is once again out of the diet. If all goes well, mark that food as safe and go on to the next food on day three. This will be enough time for many food sensitivities. However, if you have unresolved symptoms after a week, you may want to incorporate up to four days between challenge foods.

You can test foods in any order you prefer.

CHAPTER 11

Maintenance Diet

Congratulations on making it to the maintenance diet phase! You've figured out your trigger foods, and it's time to develop a longer-term eating plan. Variety is key. Make food choices that are as diverse as possible while staying away from your trigger foods. To get started, take a look at the maintenance diet food lists in Chapter 17. If you see foods that you need to eliminate, go ahead and cross them out with a red pen. If a food you love is missing and you know it's safe for you, write it down on the appropriate food list. These lists will help get you started on healthy meal planning.

The goal of the maintenance diet is to make sure you are getting a balanced diet with all the macronutrients and micronutrients you need every day from vegetables, fruit, whole grains, healthy proteins, and healthy fats. Review the daily meal guidelines in Chapter 17 for recommendations on how much to eat from each food group.

Now that you are ready to start on your maintenance diet, it's time for you to learn some basic meal planning techniques. People with food restrictions need to be careful about what they eat while getting enough nutrients and energy to support a healthy, active body and lifestyle. That's where meal planning comes in.

You'll see a step-by-step guide to creating meal plans in this chapter. It might look complex at first, but planning meals is a skill that will help you manage your health for the long term, so we will be walking through the steps in this chapter.

Do you know how to plan for a week's worth of meals and snacks so that you make only one big trip to the grocery store each week? You can plan meals for a week, a month, or anything in between. The process is simple and straight forward, and once you get used to it, it'll probably take just a few minutes each week.

Meal planning saves time and money, and the little bit of up-front work saves you from the nightly struggle of deciding what to eat. This is especially important when you are making changes to your diet, whether you are eating more vegetables, on an elimination diet, or on a maintenance diet. Meal planning is a skill that will help you beyond your experience with this book or any elimination diet. It is a life skill that makes it easier to eat right, and you can save money if meal plans are created efficiently.

Meal Planning 101

1. Create a list of all the foods you can eat. One way to start this process is to look at the food lists in Chapter 17. There are lists for protein foods, grain/starch foods, vegetables, and fruit. You can cross out any foods that you can't eat or don't like. By the same token, if you notice there are foods missing that you love and are safe for you to eat, write them down on the same food list.

2. Plan your dinners first. Figure that you will use leftovers in the next day's lunch. Plan your breakfasts last.

   a. Choose your vegetables for the week. Figure that you will eat the more perishable ingredients earlier in the week and the heartier ones later in the week. This helps you go grocery shopping only once a week. For example, in the "green" category, I'd make sure to eat butter lettuce before I broke out the kale. In the "red/orange" category, I'd eat bell peppers before carrots. Meal plans usually begin with proteins as the "center of the plate" item, but the way we think about healthy eating has changed a lot since the 1950s, and so I'm going to begin by emphasizing the most important part of your plate: vegetables. Half your plate should be devoted to them.

   b. Choose your proteins. Proteins tend to be more perishable, so think about how long they'll last when meal planning. For example, I tend to cook fish in the first couple of days of the week. Then I move on to chicken, turkey, or pork. Finally, I move on to beef. Once cooked, foods can last three to four days in the refrigerator. Sometimes I'll make a midweek run to the store to pick up a few odds and ends, maybe a fresh protein. If not, I might make legumes the protein of the day: canned chickpeas and tetra-pack black bean soup are both pantry staples for me. I may also break out canned sardines or tuna or eggs for a quick, late-week meal. Pair the proteins with the vegetables by perishability and your palate. I recommend that you choose seasonal vegetables that are safe for you to eat. Poultry and fish may go better with lightly prepared vegetables that are steamed or baked with acidic notes from citrus or vinegar; red meat may go better with vegetables that are sautéed or roasted with deeper flavors from tomatoes, mushrooms, or balsamic vinegar. These are just a few ideas; let your own tastes be your guide.

c. Choose grains or starches that will complement your vegetables and proteins. For example, if I wanted to eat asparagus early in the week, I might choose baby red potatoes as my starch. Grains and starches are usually more stable (less perishable); generally, you can enjoy them any time of the week. Pair grains or starch foods with your protein-vegetable combo. And voilà, you have a meal!

d. Vegetables, cooked proteins, and grains or starch foods can usually fit into two days of meals. They can be dinner one night and part of lunch or even dinner the next night.

3. Lunch. Some of your lunches can simply be smaller portions of the previous night's dinner. You can add a fresh fruit or vegetable.

4. Breakfast. If you're like most Americans, you don't have time for breakfast. This is an area where you may want to keep it simple. Try plain oatmeal with fruit and nuts. Or make toast with a forty-five-second microwaved egg on top and a slice of tomato. On the grocery list you'd just have to remember to buy a loaf of bread, eggs, a tomato, oatmeal, and the same fruit and nuts you'll use for snacks.

5. Snacks. Figure out where fruit fits in. It can be apple slices after dinner or chopped bananas and walnuts in your morning oatmeal. Sometimes my afternoon go-to snack of a pear and pistachios will substitute for a sit-down breakfast for me. Aim to eat a piece of fruit every day. Veggies are also great snacks. Try carrot sticks, bell peppers, and cucumber slices with dressing.

Meal Planning: Getting Started

The easiest way to do this is to use the food lists in Chapter 17: Maintenance Diet Tools and cross out any foods that are not allowed for you. Then, using these same sheets, choose only from the safe foods for you. For each meal, choose a vegetable, a protein, and a grain or starch. Add healthy fats to meals and snacks as appropriate (just don't go overboard on calories). You may choose from any of the food lists for your snacks, but it'll probably be easiest to snack on fresh fruit and nuts (if they are safe for you).

1. Go to the food lists in the maintenance diet tools. Cross out any foods that are not safe for you. Add any favorite safe foods that are missing. This is now your universe of safe foods.

Single Meal

2. For a single meal, choose a food from each group that follows. Putting them together can be as easy as doing a quick Internet search, typing in the foods and the word recipe.

Vegetable:

Protein:

Grain or starch:

Meal idea:

Weekly Meals

3. For a week of meals, it is easier to choose a handful of foods from each food list that you'd like to use that week.

   Vegetables *(choose three to five different ones, especially dark green and orange)*:

   Protein foods *(choose at least three different ones, and try to make at least one a plant protein)*:

   Grains or starches *(choose at least two different ones, and try to make at least one a whole grain)*:

4. Mix and match foods so that you always end up with a meal that has a vegetable, a protein, and a grain or starch. Use fresh fish, poultry, and delicate produce (think tender greens, summer squash, or asparagus) at the beginning of the week; use fresh pork or beef midweek through the fifth day; and use heartier vegetables throughout the week (think carrots, onions, potatoes, or winter squash). Plant proteins, such as beans, often last weeks or months, as do frozen versions of fresh meats.

Meal Planning Worksheet

	Breakfast	Lunch	Dinner	Snacks
Day 1				
Day 2				
Day 3				
Day 4				
Day 5				

	Breakfast	Lunch	Dinner	Snacks
Day 6				
Day 7				

Grocery List

5. Here are my top tips for easy meal planning:

   • Always make enough for next-day leftovers.

   • Choose a few simple foods to have on hand as snacks throughout the week.

   • Don't forget to defrost frozen meats the night before.

   • Include a vegetable or a fruit every time you eat.

   • Don't be fatphobic. Healthy fats are good for you, and add flavor and nutrition to meals.

   • Keep your pantry and freezer stocked with healthy essentials, and you'll always be ready to whip something up.

   • Consider getting a rice cooker or a slow cooker. If you'll be eating a lot of rice, a rice cooker makes it so easy to prepare. A slow cooker can make soups a cinch.

   • Go for seasonal foods. They taste better and will probably be more affordable, too.

Expert Tips on Choosing, Storing, and Preparing Fruits and Vegetables

A free online resource from the Produce for Better Health Foundation (www.fruitsandveggies morematters.org/fruit-vegetable-nutrition-database) offers a fruit and vegetable database that includes selection, storage, and nutrition information, and will also tell you what's in season. The site also has a video library with topics like eating healthy on a budget; smart snacking; kid-friendly, quick-to-fix; and more: www.fruitsandveggiesmorematters.org/video/VideoCenter.php#show_the_video_result.

• Don't feel like cooking dinner every night of the week? You'll probably have more than enough food left over to skip making dinner at least one night.

Special Feature: Resident Bacteria and Friends

It has been suggested that a healthy gut can alleviate digestive symptoms from food sensitivities, such as diarrhea and irritable bowel syndrome. While an elimination diet may be able to reset the gut so that it has a balance of foods that promotes a diverse microbiome, the maintenance diet helps establish and encourage the microbiome to flourish.

There is growing interest in how "good" gut bacteria can help keep the body healthy. However, I should start this section by stating that the following content is about an extremely young and emerging area of science. This means that we are far from having final answers on just about every question. Still, it is a very exciting area of study because of what it could mean for how we understand human health. Please read on with that caveat in mind, and stay tuned over the years for enough research saying the same thing to the point that we find ourselves with credible reliable recommendations.

The American Gut Project

The American Gut Project (www.americangut.org) wants to do for the gut what the Human Genome Project did for genes. They are crowd-sourcing data, asking for volunteers to provide data and samples in the largest open-source silent project in the world, so that they can understand the microbiota in the gut. Why are they doing this? Because they know that factors such as age, diet, family, pets, smoking, drinking, environment, and more all affect the microbiome, but they don't know which factors are most important. All this information is just the start. First, they need to understand the bacteria inside the body and how diet and lifestyle affect it. Next, they may be able to generate ideas for future health research.

Go Ahead, Use the Royal "We"

You might think of yourself as a single living being, but inside you there are about 100 trillion microorganisms (of at least 500 different types), most of them pretty harmless and probably more helpful than not. They protect the body from harmful bacteria, help with digestion, including the ability to absorb nutrients, and help the immune system stay healthy. These microorganisms are also called our resident bacteria, our microflora, our intestinal flora, and our microbiota. The universe of their genes is called the microbiome (similar to the universe of "our" genes being called the human genome).

The health of all those trillions of microorganisms is also thought to be connected to allergies; chronic inflammation; metabolic diseases, such as obesity, heart disease, and diabetes; an even mood; and more. To be clear, we don't know all the details.

Just about all scientists working in the microbiome area of research today will tell you that it's too early to draw conclusions about what it means for human health.

How do all those bugs get inside me?

It started when you were born. The gut of an infant is more or less a blank slate, and it gets most of its first bacteria through natural birth (vs. C-section) and breast-feeding. Those two things help get the new infant gut settled with a flourishing population of good resident bacteria. One of the benefits of having this good resident bacteria is that there is less room for harmful bacteria, which could damage the gut. By age three, the resident bacteria in the gut is largely established for life.

Does that mean I can't change my intestinal flora?

Once the microbiota is established, by age three, it tends to resist change. You may still be able to change your resident bacteria, but it doesn't happen easily. Antibiotics can kill off much of your microflora, leaving the door open for new bacteria to colonize the gut–good or bad. Also, changing what you eat could change the proportions of different bacteria populations in your gut. One of the ways diet can affect the microflora is through probiotics and prebiotics.

The tip of the iceberg: Prebiotics and probiotics and synbiotics

At the very tip of the iceberg of microbiome knowledge, we have the little we understand about probiotics and prebiotics and their role in health. Probiotics are the good bacteria that help maintain a healthful and natural balance of organisms throughout the digestive tract, without which bad bacteria–would have the opportunity to take over and make a person sick. More than 500 types of these good bacteria have been identified, and the healthy human body can host 10^{12} microorganisms per gram. Some probiotics are found naturally as live cultures in yogurts, some are added to foods (including yogurts), and some are available as dietary supplements. Note that only certain strains are shown to have a benefit. Probiotics are also assisted by prebiotics, which is the food that promotes the growth of probiotics. Current research is focused on the kind of fiber that we can't digest but that our probiotics can, namely oligosaccharides, and its role in health.

Why should I care about having good bacteria in my digestive system?

It has been suggested that a healthy gut can alleviate many symptoms related to food intake. An elimination diet may be able to reset the gut so that it has a balance of foods that promotes a diverse microbiome. But only certain types of bacteria or yeast (called strains) have been shown to work in the digestive tract.

It still needs to be proved which probiotics (alone or in combination) work to treat disease. At this point, even the strains of probiotics that have been proven to work for a specific disease are not widely available.

How do probiotics work?

"Work" is the operative word here, because it is the work that probiotics do for the body that makes them valuable. They have a job to do: They must produce compounds that promote human health (e.g., vitamin K and folate) if they are to qualify for the position of probiotic. (more information follows). Probiotics are found in foods such as yogurt with live and active cultures, unpasteurized sauerkraut, kimchi, miso soup, and sourdough bread. Healthy populations of probiotics leave no room for harmful bacteria. Probiotics make up the body's microflora (aka microbiota, aka good bacteria). Probiotics feed on the parts of food that the body doesn't digest, which end up in the large intestine; these parts of food are called prebiotics.

What are the more promising benefits of probiotics?

The research is strongest for the use of probiotics in reducing diarrhea, especially if it's related to antibiotics, but also if it's due to lactose intolerance. Oddly enough, this means that some types of dairy (yogurt and kefir) could help with lactose intolerance. Probiotics may also be helpful for people with chronic digestive conditions, such as inflammatory bowel diseases, including Crohn's disease and ulcerative colitis; there is also promise for irritable bowel syndrome. Probiotics might help you stay symptom-free longer, but research has not yet pointed out which probiotics work best. Probiotics may also be helpful for urinary tract infections and yeast infections, perhaps by restoring a good balance of microorganisms to that part of the body. These areas of research are still being studied.

There are theories as to how probiotics do their good work. They may work with the immune system to tweak it in ways beneficial to the body, perhaps so that it can reduce the severity of an allergic response or help shorten the duration and reduce the severity of the common cold. They may also help keep the lining of the intestines (epithelium) strong. When it's weakened, it's easier for toxins to get through the intestinal wall barrier and into the bloodstream, which can trigger a low-grade inflammation. This type of inflammation has been implicated in many chronic autoimmune conditions, including rheumatoid arthritis, asthma, inflammatory bowel diseases, heart disease, and even cancers and other diseases. Are

> ## Did you know?
>
> Breast milk helps colonize the brand new infant's digestive tract with good bacteria. Research has found that babies delivered by C-section lack the bacteria found in babies delivered vaginally, and babies fed only with formula lacked the bacteria found in those given breast milk. Having healthy amounts of and a diversity of gut bacteria may educate the immune cells about what to attack and what to leave alone (e.g., food and dust).

probiotics the answer? It is too early to tell, and we also don't know the exact effectiveness of products on the market for specific conditions.

In the meantime, a safe way to include prebiotics and probiotics is to eat them in foods where they occur naturally (whole grains, nuts, and beans contain prebiotics; probiotics may be found in foods like yogurt with live and active cultures, unpasteurized sauerkraut, kimchi, miso soup, and sourdough bread). These foods are a good fit in an overall healthful diet anyway.

What are the promising benefits of prebiotics?

Prebiotics are fuel for probiotics. Unlike probiotics—which have to be strong enough to remain alive in the harsh acids of the stomach and small intestine, surviving long enough to colonize the large intestine—prebiotics are easy to come by in the form of undigested carbohydrates (e.g., dietary fiber). Prebiotics can help the body by helping the good resident bacteria already in the gut grow in numbers and diversity.

There are hundreds of complex carbohydrates that qualify as prebiotics, including different types of fiber (e.g., soluble fiber, insoluble fiber, and resistant starch; resistant starch is another type of dietary fiber that "resists" digestion and can be found in legumes, bananas, and cooked and chilled pasta and rice), and these prebiotics are available in just about all plant foods: nuts, vegetables, fruit, and whole grains. The reason to look for prebiotics in food instead of a fiber supplement is that there is more diversity in foods, and a person needs diverse fuel for a diverse population of probiotics. Certain resident bacteria will prefer one type of fiber while a different type of resident bacteria will prefer something else. Population size, as well as diversity, of resident bacteria is important.

In the United States, fiber is already on the list of things we need to add to our diets. Most Americans aren't meeting daily recommendations for fiber. Today, fiber isn't recommended because of what it does for our microbiota. There are plenty of other reasons to increase fiber intake, including relieving constipation; keeping the bowels healthy and free of pouches; preventing hemorrhoids; lowering cholesterol (the job of soluble fiber, found in beans, oats, and flax); improving blood sugar levels; and promoting a healthy weight (through longer chewing times and by providing more nutrients than refined grains). The idea that eating a variety of different fibers can help with microbiota diversity is just an added perk.

Prebiotics are thought to have multiple benefits, from improving the makeup of gut microbiota to promoting regularity and even better bone health through better calcium absorption. Prebiotics may also support the GI system to create substances the body needs for normal metabolism, satiety, and immunity. Prebiotics may also have a role in reducing the risk of intestinal infections, reduce the risk and improve the symptoms of intestinal inflammation, and very preliminary findings suggest they may have a role in reducing the risk of obesity, type 2 diabetes, and metabolic syndrome, though it's not well understood how. One theory is that because prebiotics promote growth of good bacteria, that then compete with harmful bacteria, that a decline in healthy bacteria could lead to low-grade inflammation linked with metabolic diseases such as obesity.

How do prebiotics work?

Prebiotics are basically food for probiotics. They help probiotics multiply and help the gut stay healthy. Most of the current research on prebiotics looks at certain carbohydrates (oligosaccharides) that remain undigested until they make it to the large intestine and probiotics consume them. The most common prebiotics on the market in the United States are inulin fructans and fructo-oligosaccharides (FOS). They work by providing fuel for probiotics, which then multiply and flourish in order to benefit the body. Some prebiotics are shown to help increase calcium absorption. They may also play a role—per experimental animal and human studies—in helping with satiety and thus healthy weight.

Why do I want lots of microorganisms inside me to be well fed?

Keeping the good bugs well fed and flourishing means less room and an unwelcoming environment for bacteria that could be harmful. Your resident bacteria also produce all kinds of things that you need: enzymes, vitamins, neurotransmitters, and signaling molecules that affect the immune system and metabolism.

Probiotics keep the digestive tract healthy. They break down food that the body can't, such as some dietary fibers (this and any other fuel for the probiotics are called prebiotics). As a side effect of probiotics chowing down on the food we don't digest, they create important micronutrients for the body, such as vitamin K, biotin, thiamine, vitamin B12, and folate. When you have good neighbors, there just isn't room for bad ones. Probiotics work in much the same way. With a healthy population of probiotics, the bacteria that cause disease have nowhere to colonize. When you stop using your muscles, you tend to lose them. In much the same way, probiotics and the immune system in the digestive tract have a good working relationship, and the constant conversations they have keep the gut immune system healthy and prepared to fight bacteria that are actually harmful when the time comes.

What about those probiotics I see on TV commercials? Should I buy them?

You may be referring to certain commercials for yogurt that tout their probiotics (live and active cultures). When probiotics and prebiotics are combined in the same food, that food is called a synbiotic (e.g., yogurt with live and active cultures that has fiber added to it). The body needs to be exposed to both probiotics and prebiotics on a regular basis to change the microflora. Otherwise, the body's gut tends to go back to its original makeup of microorganisms.

OK, so what do probiotics have to do with food sensitivities?

There is a lot we are still learning about probiotics, and this is an exciting emerging area of research. That said, there is encouraging evidence that probiotics can help with digestive issues that may be linked to food sensitivities, such as diarrhea and irritable bowel syndrome. Although we don't have all the answers, because these foods are healthful, they can be incorporated into the maintenance diet.

PART FOUR
Tools to Help You

CHAPTER 12

Getting Started

These worksheets will be helpful during the assessment phase before you begin the elimination diet. Fill them out as thoroughly as possible to set yourself up for success.

Initial Food Sensitivity Profile

Name:	
Sex:	Age:

What foods do you eat most often?

What foods will be hardest to give up?

What medications do you take regularly and what are they for?

What conditions are you already diagnosed with (e.g., high blood pressure, anxiety, and so on)?

Do you have any nonfood allergies, for example, allergies to pollen, mold spores, dust, animal dander, bug bites, perfume, or smoke?

What are your symptoms?

Take stock of your symptoms and rate them on a scale of 1 to 5, with 1 being mild and 5 being severe. You'll track your symptoms throughout this journey and come back to these baseline values to see what kind of progress you've made. Following is a list of symptoms that people have reported in connection with food intolerances and allergies. If you have a symptom that is not on the list, write it down and keep track of it throughout the elimination diet.

- Bloating
- Congestion
- Cramps
- Diarrhea
- Eczema
- Gas
- Headaches
- Hives

- Irritability
- Itchy ear canal
- Itchy mouth
- Itchy skin (elsewhere)
- Nausea
- Nervousness
- Odd taste in mouth

- Redness of skin around the eyes
- Runny nose
- Slight, dry cough
- Sneezing
- Stomach pain
- Uterine contractions
- Vomiting

How long have you been experiencing your symptoms overall (e.g., weeks, months, or years)?

What food causes your symptoms, and has this food caused these symptoms more than once?

How much of the food did you eat when the symptoms occurred?

Was the food cooked on the stovetop, baked in the oven, or raw?

How long after you were exposed to the food did your symptoms occur?

Have you ever eaten the food without these symptoms occurring?

Were other factors involved, such as exercise, alcohol, or the use of aspirin or nonsteroidal anti-inflammatory drugs?

Have you had these symptoms other than after being exposed to the food?

What treatment did you receive, and how long did the symptoms last?

Have you ever had or been diagnosed with an inhalant allergy (pollen, mold spores, dust, animal dander), food allergy, food additive intolerance, allergy to bug bites, or any other allergies?

The following symptoms are more severe, and if you are experiencing any of these, seek medical attention:

- Swelling of lips, tongue, or throat
- Trouble swallowing
- Shortness of breath or wheezing

- Turning blue
- Drop in blood pressure (feeling faint, confused, or weak; passing out)
- Loss of consciousness

- Chest pain
- Weakened pulse
- Sense of impending doom

Self-Efficacy Worksheet

My goal is the following:
I am going on the elimination diet because I believe it will help me in this way:
Here is what I am willing to do to reach my goal:
On a scale of 1 to 10, my confidence that I can do this is as follows:
On a scale of 1 to 10, the level of importance to me to do this is as follows:

Kitchen Checklist

Prepare your kitchen by setting aside dedicated tools with which to prepare food, cook it, and eat it during the elimination diet. Following is a basic starter guide for the materials you will want to set aside.

Storage Area

You'll need a home for your personal kitchen items while you're on the elimination diet. Make arrangements with your household, and find a space that will fit everything while also being separate enough to be safe from cross-contamination. In other words, keep your things away from open areas that could be splashed by others' cooking, Also, keep your things above areas where food is stored.

Cooking Preparation and Tools

Kitchen tools and utensils:

  1 mixing bowl made of glass or aluminum (if you have them to spare, you may want to set aside 2 or 3 for yourself, as they come in handy in the kitchen while cooking)

  2 cutting boards, one for plants and one for meats

  1 all-purpose knife (no need to purchase a whole new knife set)

  1 mixing spoon

  1 spatula

  1 food thermometer

  1 food processor

Cooking vessels:

  1 medium pot made of aluminum or iron

  1 cast-iron frying pan

Dinnerware:

  1 drinking glass

  1 hot beverage mug

  1 plate

  1 bowl

  1 fork, knife, and spoon; chopsticks

CHAPTER 13

Targeted Elimination Diet

If you have negative reactions to fewer than five foods on the allowed foods list on page 126, the Targeted Elimination Diet is the plan for you. (Although the number five is somewhat arbitrary; do what feels best for you.) This four-week diet plan can be used to target just one food type, or you can select a handful of food types, such as a few of the eight major allergens, or other additives like tartrazine, MSG, benozates, or sulfites. (If you're experiencing reactions to a greater number of foods, you might consider the Catchall Elimination Diet, beginning on page 144).

Follow the basic steps of the elimination diet outlined earlier in this book: assess, plan, avoid, challenge, maintain. The following worksheets and charts will help you plan your meals while on the diet, as well as help track any symptoms you may have.

Assess: Food and Symptom Tracker

The first time you keep a food and symptom tracker will be in the assessment phase, before you start the elimination diet. Keep your diet as close to your regular routine as possible. The idea is to record your typical diet, so you can see what veering away from it in the weeks that follow will do to how you feel.

Every time you eat or drink something, be sure you're answering these five questions, and of course, record the time your symptoms start and stop:

1. What is it?

2. What's in it?

3. How much did I eat?

4. How do I feel?

5. Is there anything else going on?

Following is an example of a journal you can use to track your symptoms. Some sample entries are provided.

Sample Food and Symptom Tracker

Meal	Food/Drink (How Much)	Ingredients	Symptoms
Breakfast Time:	8 oz orange juice 1 Tbsp dry oatmeal with ½ cup hot water	Orange juice, calcium Oatmeal, tap water	Symptoms: Start time: End time: Rating:
AM Snack Time:	23 almonds 1 medium nectarine	Almonds Nectarine	Symptoms: Start time: End time: Rating:
Lunch Time:	1 chicken taco	1 6-inch all natural corn tortilla (corn, water, lime, salt), grilled chicken, coleslaw (cabbage, onion, lime juice, salt, and pepper), salsa (tomatoes, onion, cilantro, lime juice, and salt)	Symptoms: Start time: End time: Rating:
PM Snack Time:			Symptoms: Start time: End time: Rating:

Meal	Food/Drink (How Much)	Ingredients	Symptoms
Dinner Time:			Symptoms: Start time: End time: Rating:
PM Snack Time:			Symptoms: Start time: End time: Rating:
Notes: Make a note of anything else that's going on that you think could be affecting how your body reacts whether it's stress; premenstrual syndrome (PMS); being around animals, gardens, or moldy places; having a cold; or even enjoying a hard workout.			

Plan: Prep Your Pantry for Targeted Elimination Diet

Pantry Favorites

- Black beans (dry or canned)

- Brown rice

- Buckwheat groats

- Buckwheat noodles (100 percent buckwheat, not a wheat and buckwheat blend)

- Canned beans of any variety

- Garbanzo beans (chickpeas) (dry or canned)

- Gluten-free pasta

- Lentils (dry)

- Olive oil, canola oil

- Pepper

- Quinoa

- Rice milk

- Rice noodles

- Split peas (dry)

- Sea salt

- Wild rice

Other pantry foods to choose from:

Plant protein: Black-eyed peas, lima beans, navy beans, pinto beans white beans. Choose dry beans when possible; if not, check label ingredients carefully to avoid any additives and preservatives.

Plant milks: Brown rice milk, hemp milk, oat milk, potato milk

Oils and seasonings: canola oil, flaxseed oil, grapeseed oil, Olive oil, safflower oil, sunflower oil, salt, black pepper, white pepper

Plain starches are safest: Amaranth, buckwheat, cassava, chickpea, cornmeal, corn on the cob, millet, oats, popcorn, potatoes, quinoa, rice, tapioca, teff, wild rice

These packaged foods are likely OK, but still check the label: Brown rice pasta, corn pasta, cream of rice, mung bean pasta, oat bran, oatmeal, puffed amaranth, puffed millet, puffed rice, rice flakes, rolled oats, quinoa flakes, quinoa pasta, wild rice pasta, plain rice cakes, and rice crackers without any forbidden ingredients, dried fruit that is specifically sulfite-free

Fresh Favorites

- Apples
- Bananas
- Beef
- Broccoli
- Butternut squash
- Celery
- Zucchini
- Chicken
- Cucumbers
- Green beans
- Kale
- Pears
- Yams

Other fresh foods to choose from:

Vegetables: Artichokes, arugula, asparagus, Belgian endive, bell peppers, bok choy, broccoflower, broccolini, Brussels sprouts, butter lettuce, cabbage, cauliflower, collard greens, dark green leafy lettuce, garlic, iceberg lettuce, jicama, kabocha squash, leeks, mesclun, mustard greens, okra, onions, parsnips, radish, red peppers, romaine lettuce, shallots, snow peas, sugar snap peas, summer squash, Swiss chard, turnip greens, turnips, watercress

Starchy Vegetables: Acorn squash, beets, carrots, corn, crookneck squash, French beans, green lima beans, Hubbard squash, plantains, sweet potatoes, whole potatoes, green peas

Fruit: Asian pears, cantaloupe, figs, guava, honeydew melon, kiwifruit, lemons, limes, mangoes, mangosteen, persimmons, pineapples, pomegranates, star fruit, watermelons

Animal protein: Pork, turkey

Herbs: basil, cilantro, oregano, parsley, rosemary

Food Allowed on the Targeted Elimination Diet

Vegetables	
What you can eat	Most plain, minimally processed (nothing added) fresh and frozen vegetables
Do not eat	Soybeans, soybean sprouts, sprouted wheat, mixed sprouts, red beans, pumpkin, spinach, tomatoes, sliced potatoes, mushrooms, frozen potatoes
Foods to eat	**Dark green** Bok choy, broccoli, collard greens, dark green leafy lettuce, kale, mesclun, mustard greens, romaine lettuce, turnip greens, watercress, arugula, Belgian endive, broccoflower, broccolini **Starchy** Black-eyed peas, green peas, french beans, green lima beans, plantains, whole potatoes, corn, yams **Red and orange** Acorn squash, butternut squash, carrots, Hubbard squash, red peppers, sweet potatoes **Beans and peas** Black beans, black-eyed peas (dry), garbanzo beans (chickpeas), lentils, navy beans, pinto beans, split peas, white beans, crookneck squash **Other** Artichokes, asparagus, beets, Brussels sprouts, cabbage, cauliflower, celery, cucumbers, green beans, bell peppers, iceberg lettuce, okra, onions, garlic, turnips, zucchini, jicama, sugar snap peas, snow peas, shallots, kabocha squash, leeks, parsnips, radish, acorn squash, butter lettuce, butternut squash, summer squash Swiss chard
Notes	Aim for 2.5 cups a day, especially green and orange vegetables.
Fruits	
What you can eat	Most plain, whole, fresh, and frozen fruits
Do not eat	Grapes, berries (e.g., strawberries, cranberries, raspberries), stone fruits (apricots, cherries, plums, prunes, peaches, nectarine, avocados), oranges, grapefruit, papayas, tomatoes
Foods to eat	Apples, persimmons, kiwifruit, bananas, mangoes, pears, pineapple, cantaloupe, honeydew melons, watermelons, Asian pears, figs, guava, star fruit, mangosteen Lemons, limes Dried fruit that is specifically sulfite-free Pomegranates
Notes	Aim for 2 cups a day

Grains/Starches	
What you can eat	Plain, unbleached versions of gluten-free, wheat-free grains are safest. Packaged plain cereals, pastas, and crackers made from safe grains are likely OK, but be sure to double-check the label for any forbidden ingredients.
Do not eat	Be aware of grain mixes or any products with multiple ingredients.
Foods to eat	Plain grains and starches are safest: amaranth, buckwheat, chickpea, millet, teff, oats, potatoes, quinoa, rice, wild rice, tapioca, cassava, cornmeal, corn on the cob, popcorn Packaged foods that are likely OK, but still check the label: cream of rice, puffed rice, rice flakes, oatmeal, rolled oats, oat bran, puffed amaranth, puffed millet, quinoa flakes, brown rice pasta, wild rice pasta, mung bean pasta, 100% buckwheat noodles, rice noodles, quinoa pasta, corn pasta Plain rice cakes and rice crackers without any forbidden ingredients
Notes	Aim for 6 oz a day of mostly whole grains.
Protein	
What you can eat	Plain, pure, and fresh versions of meat or poultry Most plain legumes Packaged foods that are likely OK, but still check the label: egg-free egg substitutes, canned beans
Do not eat	Soybeans, peanuts
Foods to eat	Chicken, turkey, pork, beef, split peas, black beans, black-eyed peas, garbanzo beans (chickpeas), lentils, lima beans, navy beans, pinto beans, split peas, white beans
Notes	Aim for 5.5 oz per day of mostly plant protein
Dairy Substitute	
What you can eat	Plain, plant-based milks. These are sometimes fortified with calcium and vitamin D.
Do not eat	Flavored milks
Foods to eat	Rice milk, brown rice milk, oat milk, potato milk, hemp milk
Notes	Aim for 3 cups per day, and consider a calcium and vitamin D supplement.
Oils	
What you can eat	Certain vegetable oils
Do not eat	Peanut oil, tree nut oils, soybean oil, any oil with hydrolyzed lecithin
Foods to eat	Olive oil, canola oil, sunflower oil, safflower oil, flaxseed oil, grapeseed oil

Beverages	
What you can eat	Water
Foods to eat	Water
Notes	Let your urine be your guide as to how much water you drink: it should be light yellow; don't let yourself get thirsty. Water and other food sources all count toward hydration, so sticking to the 8 cups per day rule of thumb for water should suffice.
Herbs and Spices	
What you can eat	Salt and pepper
Do not eat	Most herbs, spices, sweeteners
Foods to eat	Salt, black pepper, white pepper Herbs: parsley, basil, oregano, rosemary, cilantro

Foods by Perishability

Creating meal plans can be challenging even without food restrictions, but the process is the same. You start with a set of foods and mix and match to create meals and snacks, being sure to use up the more perishable foods earlier in the week. Here, I've created weekly meal plans to take some of the work out of your elimination diet. The week starts on Saturday, when you are more likely to have time to cook. I have provided meal plans for the Targeted Elimination Diet (free of all major allergens and processed foods).

Food Guide by Perishability for the Targeted Elimination Diet

High Perishability use up in 1 to 2 days		
Vegetables	**Fruit**	**Animal Protein**
Arugula	Figs	Chicken
Corn on the cob	Mangosteen	Turkey
Okra	Pineapple	
Swiss chard	Plantains, ripe	
Sugar snap peas		
Turnip greens		
Turnips		

Medium Perishability use up in 3 to 5 days				
Vegetables		**Fruit**		**Animal Protein**
Asparagus	Kale	Cantaloupe (once opened)		Beef
Bell peppers	Mustard greens	Guava		Pork
Broccoflower	Red peppers	Mangoes		
Broccoli	Romaine lettuce	Persimmon		
Broccoli rabe	Snow peas	Watermelon (once opened)		
Butter lettuce	Summer squash			
Cauliflower	Sweet potatoes			
Collard greens	Watercress			
Green peas	Zucchini			
Low Perishability use up anytime in the week				
Acorn squash	Garlic	Apples		
Beets	Green beans	Asian pears		
Artichokes	Iceberg lettuce	Bananas		
Belgian endive	Jicama	Honeydew		
Bok choy	Leeks	Kiwifruit		
Broccolini	Onions	Lemons		
Brussels sprouts	Parsnips	Limes		
Cabbage	Potatoes, whole	Pears		
Carrots	Radish	Star fruit		
Celery	Shallots			
Cucumbers	Squash (butternut, crookneck, Hubbard, kabocha)			
Dark green leafy lettuce				
French beans	Yam			
Pantry and Freezer Staples lasts a week or longer				
Vegetables and Fruit		**Grains** (plain are safest)*		**Animal Protein**
Black beans	Peas, frozen	Amaranth	Popcorn	Frozen chicken
Black-eyed peas	Lentils	Buckwheat	Quinoa	Frozen turkey
Corn, frozen	Navy beans	Cassava	Rice	Frozen pork
Dried fruit that is specifically sulfite-free	Pinto beans	Chickpea	Tapioca	Frozen beef
	Split peas	Cornmeal	Teff	
Garbanzo beans (chickpeas)	White beans	Millet	Wild rice	
Green lima beans, frozen		Oats		

*In addition to plain grains, there may be safe packaged foods. These are likely OK, but still check the label: Cream of rice, puffed rice, rice flakes, oatmeal, rolled oats, oat bran, puffed amaranth, puffed millet, quinoa flakes, brown rice pasta, wild rice pasta, mung bean pasta, 100% buckwheat noodles, rice noodles, quinoa pasta, corn pasta, plain rice cakes and rice crackers without any forbidden ingredients

Plant Milks and Water	Oils	Herbs & Spices
Rice milk	Canola oil	Basil
Brown rice milk	Flaxseed oil	Black pepper
Oat milk	Grapeseed oil	Cilantro
Potato milk	Olive oil	Oregano
Hemp milk	Sunflower oil	Parsley
Water	Safflower oil	Rosemary
		Salt
		White pepper

Eliminate: Begin Your Targeted Elimination Diet

Take some of the work out of your Targeted Elimination Diet by using the two weeks of meals plans provided here. You can also use the blank template on page 143 to create your own meal plans.

Week 1 Meal Plan for the Targeted Elimination Diet

	Breakfast	Lunch/Dinner	Lunch/Dinner	Snacks
Monday	Oatmeal made with rice milk and topped with apples	Butternut squash and apple soup with ground turkey and onion With freshly cut apple slices	Pork loin Wild rice with sweet potato Steamed broccolini	
Tuesday	Small serving of butternut squash soup	Pork loin chopped with wild rice sweet potato, and shredded Brussels sprouts	Beef cubes, roasted Brussels sprouts, onions, and carrots	Sweet potato rounds
Wednesday	Baked sweet potato and apples	Beef cubes over wild rice medley	Easy midweek meal Brown rice penne pasta with pesto and leftover broccolini	Carrot sticks
Thursday	Fruit and Veggie smoothie with any leftovers. Bananas and apples make a great smoothie starter; add leafy greens, cucumbers, fresh parsley, oat milk, and ice cubes.	Leftover pasta with pesto	Stuffed bell pepper stuffed with medley of chickpeas, onion, garlic, zucchini, quinoa, apple	Apples
Friday	Day 2 fruit & Veggie smoothie (toss anything that hasn't been consumed by the end of day 2)	Chickpea-quinoa medley; enjoy as a hearty dip with rice crackers or on cucumber slices	"Kitchen Sink Fried Rice" with brown rice and remaining vegetables, chopped	Steamed artichoke with olive oil and lemon dipping sauce
Saturday	Brown rice porridge made with rice milk, topped with very ripe bananas or mangoes	Butternut squash and apple soup with ground turkey and onion With rice crackers	Grilled chicken with basil-garlic pesto, sautéed zucchini, roasted red potatoes	Sugar snap peas

	Breakfast	Lunch/Dinner	Lunch/Dinner	Snacks
Prep	Save some chicken, pesto, and soup for tomorrow Save leftover pesto in ice cube trays, covered in freezer			
Sunday	Breakfast quinoa porridge with fresh figs	Chicken over butter lettuce, cucumbers, and rice noodles, dressed in basil pesto	Butternut squash and apple soup with ground turkey and onion With side of steamed broccoli, drizzled with extra virgin olive oil	Rice crackers

Week 1 Grocery List

Pantry (you may already have)

- Brown rice, oatmeal, quinoa, wild rice

- Chickpeas

- Rice crackers

- Rice milk or oat milk

- Rice noodles

Perishable (buy fresh)

- *Fruit*: Apples, bananas (or mangoes), fresh figs

- *Vegetables*: Artichoke, basil, bell pepper, broccolini, Brussels sprouts, butter lettuce, butternut squash, carrots, cucumbers, onion, parsley, red potatoes, sugar snap peas, sweet potato, zucchini

- *Meat*: Beef, chicken, ground turkey, pork loin

Week 2 Meal Plan for Targeted Elimination Diet

More vegetarian recipes this week, so that there are options for everyone

	Breakfast	Lunch/Dinner	Lunch/Dinner	Snacks
Monday	Fruit smoothie: get rid of any leftover fruit salad, or make a new smoothie with your choice of fruit	Kale-quinoa salad with Asian pears, onion, parsley Potato and pea soup	Easy weeknight meal: Easy red lentil soup With basic roasted cauliflower	Fruit salad
Tuesday	Oatmeal with bananas	Easy red lentil soup with carrots, onion, celery; and rice crackers	Black bean, corn, onion, cilantro tacos with organic corn tortillas with shredded green cabbage slaw	Jicama matchsticks
Prep	Thaw lean ground turkey			
Wednesday	Small serving of red lentil soup	Black beans, corn, onion, cilantro tacos with organic corn tortillas with shredded green cabbage slaw	Spaghetti squash topped with sautéed ground turkey, onion, garlic mix Fresh chopped side salad with chopped bell peppers, cucumbers, radishes, and snow peas	Kale chips
Thursday	Breakfast millet with simmered pears and pineapples	Spaghetti squash topped with sautéed ground turkey, onion, garlic mix Fresh chopped side salad with chopped bell peppers, cucumbers, radishes, and snow peas	Black bean and corn soup, served with a half-ear of corn on the cob	Carrot sticks, cucumber rounds
Friday	Cantaloupe cubes,	Black bean and corn soup, served with a half-ear of corn on the cob	Easy weeknight meal: Quinoa pasta with asparagus, olive oil, and lemon	Asian pear
Saturday	Shredded potato pancakes with apples	Pasta primavera with 100% buckwheat noodles, parsley, cauliflower, broccoli, asparagus, zucchini, fresh peas, red onion, olive oil, and lemon	White bean soup with kale, okra, and pork	Cauliflower, broccoli
Sunday	Mixed fruit of your choice from allowed fruit list (depending on what's in season, try fresh figs, banana, and apples; or watermelon, cantaloupe, and honeydew; or mangoes, pineapple, and kiwifruit)	White bean soup with kale, okra, and pork	Kale-quinoa salad with Asian pears, onion, parsley Potato and pea soup	Asparagus, zucchini, fresh peas

Week 2 Grocery List

Pantry (you may already have)

- Oatmeal, millet, quinoa

- Red lentils, black beans, white beans

- Buckwheat noodles, quinoa pasta, organic corn tortillas

- Olive oil

- Rice crackers

Perishable (buy fresh)

- *Fruit*: Apples, Asian pears, bananas, cantaloupe, lemon, pears, pineapples, additional fresh seasonal fruit (your pick: apples, banana, cantaloupe, figs, honeydew, kiwifruit, mangoes, pineapple, watermelon, and so on)

- *Vegetable*: asparagus, bell peppers, broccoli, carrots, cauliflower, celery, cilantro, corn on the cob, cucumbers, fresh peas, garlic, green cabbage, kale, okra, parsley, potatoes, radishes, red onion, snow peas, spaghetti squash, zucchini

- *Meat*: Pork, ground turkey

Recipes for the Targeted Elimination Diet

Grilled Chicken with Basil-Garlic Pesto

Grilled chicken is a snap and super healthy. And pesto is simple and delicious, plus you can save leftovers in ice cube trays and use them for recipes later in the following days and weeks. According to the Food Lover's Companion, a pesto is made with fresh basil, garlic, pine nuts, Parmesan or pecorino cheese, and olive oil. However, pestos can actually be made with any of a number of herbs, and we can adapt the classic ingredients to make it elimination diet friendly. Servings: 4

Grilled Chicken

2 or 3 chicken breasts

Salt

2–4 cloves garlic

1 Tbsp olive oil

Pesto

2 cups fresh basil leaves, rinsed and stems removed (No basil around? You can use cilantro, parsley, mint, spinach, or a mix of these)

2–4 cloves of garlic

½ cup extra virgin olive oil

Salt and pepper

Grilled Chicken

1. Dry chicken breasts and then rub with salt and let rest at room temperature.

2. Meanwhile, smash garlic (or use a garlic press), and mix with olive oil (alternatively, you can blend these together in a food processor).

3. Start a pan on medium-high heat.

4. Drizzle the oil-garlic mixture evenly over the chicken breasts, and do another round of rubbing.

5. Put the chicken in the pan, and cook for 2–4 minutes on each side until done (inside must be 165 degrees F according to a meat thermometer).

6. Remove from heat and set aside.

Pesto

1. Combine basil and garlic in a food processor, and process for a few seconds until roughly combined.

2. Add olive oil slowly with the food processor going until ingredients are well combined.

3. Add salt and pepper to taste.

4. Drizzle over finished grilled chicken (it's also great over sautéed vegetables, buckwheat pasta, or spaghetti squash).

5. Pour any leftovers into an ice cube tray, and cover with plastic wrap as tightly as possible.

Chopped Pork Loin with Wild Rice, Sweet Potato, and Shredded Brussels Sprouts

This dish is great any time of year, but with its rich textures and deep flavors are perfect on a cool, brisk day in fall. Wild rice is earthy and strong enough to stand up to the flavor of Brussels sprouts, sweet potato has that satisfying mouthfeel and touch of sweetness that complements the pork. Servings: 4

2 cups wild rice, dry

1 Tbsp olive oil

3 medium sweet potatoes, washed and cubed

Salt and pepper to taste

1 Tbsp canola oil

1–2 lbs pork loin, cut into 1-inch cubes

1 cup Brussels sprouts, shredded

Fresh herbs to taste (optional)

¼ cup extra virgin olive oil

Salt and pepper to taste

1. Preheat oven to 425 degrees F.

2. Rinse wild rice 2 or 3 times with cold water. If you have a rice cooker, follow the guidelines for how much water to add to 2 cups of wild rice. If you don't have a rice cooker, combine 2 cups of wild rice with 4 cups of water in a medium pot and set heat to high. Cover tightly with a lid (if you have a clean kitchen towel, you can place it between the pot and the lid for a tighter seal). Once it boils, turn the temperature to low, and let it simmer for 45–60 minutes (take a peek at around 45 minutes, and taste-test to see if it's done). Drain any remaining liquid. Fluff with a fork and then cover until ready to eat.

3. While rice is simmering, combine the 1 Tbsp olive oil and sweet potatoes until sweet potatoes are coated, add salt and pepper if desired, and then roast in the oven for about 20 minutes. You may want to check on the sweet potatoes about halfway through and give them a stir.

4. While both the rice is simmering and your sweet potatoes are roasting, add canola oil to a sauté pan, and set on medium-high heat. Pat dry the pork loin with a paper towel, and rub with salt and pepper. Chop into cubes. Add cubes to hot sauté pan and cook, uncovered, turning occasionally, until done (approximately 8–10 minutes, or until internal temperature reaches 145 degrees F). Remove from heat and let rest.

5. Wash Brussels sprouts and herbs (if using). Trim rough stems of Brussels sprouts, and remove any wilting outer leaves. Slice Brussels sprouts in half, and then cut each half in thin ribbons. If you have a food processor, just toss the washed and trimmed Brussels sprouts in until roughly shredded. Similarly chop any herbs you're using.

6. In a large bowl, combine cooked rice, roasted sweet potatoes, sautéed pork cubes, and shredded Brussels sprouts and herbs (if using). Pour the ¼ cup olive oil over mixture, and toss to combine. Add salt and pepper to taste. Enjoy!

7. Store any leftovers in a covered container in the refrigerator.

Steamed Artichoke with Olive Oil and Lemon Dipping Sauce

A simply steamed artichoke is a beautiful thing. Servings: 1 to 2

½ lemon, cut into slices

1 clove garlic

1 artichoke

1 Tbsp olive oil

Juice from other ½ lemon

Salt and pepper to taste

1. Choose a medium pot with a lid, and put an inch or two of water in it. Add lemon slices and garlic. Cover with a steamer basket. Water should not rise through the steamer basket; if it does, pour out some of the water. Set the pot on medium-high heat to bring water to a boil. Then lower heat to a simmer.

2. Meanwhile, slice about an inch off the top of the artichoke as well as any excess stem beyond about an inch of stem.

3. Trim the thorns on the ends of the leaves with kitchen scissors.

4. Place the artichoke into the pot with the cut side down and cover. Let the artichoke steam in simmering water for about 30 minutes. It's done when the leaves come off easily.

5. Combine olive oil and lemon juice with salt and pepper to taste.

6. Peel off one leaf at a time, dip into olive oil–lemon dipping sauce, and scrape soft "meat" with teeth. Repeat. Enjoy! (Some of the bottom leaves may be tougher; just remove those and go for the more tender leaves that seem to have more "meat" on them.)

White Bean Soup with Kale, Okra, and Pork

This soup can be anything you want it to be—as long as you're using "allowed" ingredients. It's a matter of combining great fresh ingredients and letting their flavors meld until you have a savory, satisfying one-pot meal. Meat isn't necessary and you can easily omit it from the recipe to make this a vegetarian stew. Or you can substitute different meats or different vegetables for different flavor profiles. Enjoy! Servings: 4

1 Tbsp olive oil

1 small onion, chopped

Salt, to taste

Pepper, to taste

1 lb pork loin, cut in 1-inch cubes (can substitute chicken or beef if desired)

4 cups water or vegetable stock

1 bunch kale, tough stems removed and leaves chopped or torn

5–10 okra, sliced into rounds

Optional add-ins: Chopped celery, carrots

15-oz can white beans, rinsed

Olive oil, for drizzling (optional)

Salt, for sprinkling at end (optional)

Freshly ground black pepper (optional)

1. Place a large pot on medium-high heat. Add olive oil and onion, and sauté until onion turns brown and smells slightly sweet. Sprinkle with salt and pepper to taste.

2. Pat pork dry, dry rub with salt, and then cut into cubes. Brown pork cubes for a few minutes until just cooked, about 3 minutes. Remove from pot.

3. Add water (or vegetable stock), bring to a boil, and then reduce heat to simmer.

4. While water is coming to a boil, wash and chop kale and okra, add to pot, and let simmer for about 5 minutes. Add any other optional add-in vegetables at this stage as well.

5. Add white beans and cooked pork, and let simmer to combine flavors for another few minutes. Make sure pork is cooked to 145 degrees F. Taste soup. For more concentrated flavor, let simmer until it is your desired consistency and flavor. Enjoy!

6. If desired, drizzle olive oil and salt on top of soup in bowl just before eating. Adding salt at the end makes it easier to taste and can be a way to add a lot of flavor without a lot of salt. You may also want to crack fresh pepper over your soup.

Quinoa Pasta with Asparagus, Olive Oil, and Lemon

This is a simple weeknight meal.   Servings: 4

1 lb quinoa pasta

1 bunch slender asparagus, washed, with tough ends trimmed

Ice water

¼ cup olive oil

Juice from 1 lemon

Salt and pepper, to taste (optional)

1. Prepare quinoa pasta according to instructions.

2. Fill medium pot halfway with water and bring to a boil. Add asparagus to boiling water and cook for 2–4 minutes uncovered.

3. While water is coming to a boil, set aside a medium bowl and fill it with ice water.

4. Remove asparagus from boiling water, and immediately plunge it into the ice water for a minute or so before draining and gently drying asparagus with paper towels. Cut asparagus into 1-inch pieces.

5. Toss pasta, asparagus, olive oil, and juice from one lemon for a simple and satisfying meal. Season with salt and pepper if desired.

Challenge: Your Challenge Foods from Eliminated Food Groups

Note: An unsupervised open food challenge is not appropriate for anyone who has ever had an anaphylactic reaction.

Many of the symptoms of food sensitivities, although uncomfortable, are not severe, which makes an at-home open challenge OK for most people. The idea is to reintroduce a food that causes a bad reaction (not foods that cause dangerously severe reactions). An open food challenge can take the better part of a day, so make sure you set aside enough time.

Start with a small amount of the challenge food, waiting and watching for symptoms, and then repeat the process with a greater amount of the food until the symptoms appear or you've doubled a regular serving. Other than the challenge food, you should stay on an elimination diet during and between all the food challenges.

Once challenge foods are determined to be safe, add them to a list of safe foods, but keep them out of your diet until all the food challenges are done. Do this to keep the results clean. The following worksheets will help to make the process simple and organized.

For more information about the food challenges see Chapter 10.

Milk: lactose-free milk vs rice milk

Eggs: whole eggs vs egg-free egg substitute

Wheat: whole wheat pasta vs rice noodles

Soy: soy milk vs rice milk

Tree Nuts: almonds, walnuts, pistachios, cashews, hazelnuts, macadamia nuts, pine nuts

Peanuts: peanuts or peanut butter

Fish: salmon, tilapia, tuna, cod

Shellfish: shrimp, crab, lobster, crayfish

Sulfites: dried fruit with sulfites vs. dried fruit without sulfites

Benzoates: pear slices with cinnamon vs pear slices without cinnamon

Benzoates: strawberries vs apples

Tartrazine (FD&C Yellow #5, Yellow No. 5, Yellow 5): fruit punch with Yellow 5 vs 100 percent fruit juice

MSG: turkey sprinkled with MSG vs turkey without MSG

Lactose: regular milk vs lactose-free milk

Open Food Challenge Worksheet

Challenge food: _____

How much would you normally consume in a day? _____

Divide by 4: _X_

- Test 1 amount: _1/2X_

- Test 2 amount: _X_

- Test 3 amount: _2X_

- Test 4 amount: _4X_

- Test 5 amount: _8X_

For example, if you are challenging with milk, and you normally drink an 8-oz glass of milk a day, you would fill in the blanks like this:

- Challenge food: _Milk_

- How much would you normally consume in a day? _8 oz_

- Divide by 4: _2 oz_

- Test 1 amount: _1 oz_

- Test 2 amount: _2 oz_

- Test 3 amount: _4 oz_

- Test 4 amount: _8 oz_

- Test 5 amount: _16 oz_

As soon as you react to a food, make a note of it and stop the food challenge. Then follow directions for outcome 2, which follows.

At the end of the challenge, please check one of these boxes:

[   ] Outcome 1: This food is safe for me!

This is great news. However, still keep this food out of the diet for the rest of the challenge phase to keep the results clear.

[   ] Outcome 2: This food caused symptoms.

If this is the case, go back to the elimination diet for as long as it takes for symptoms to resolve, whether that's one day or seven (or more). Once symptoms have cleared up, wait an additional two days before going on to the next challenge.

Open Food Challenge Worksheet

Day 1   date: _____

Time	How Long	What to Do	Notes/Symptoms
	2 minutes	Put food on lower lip.	
	30 minutes	Monitor for a reaction. If there are no symptoms, proceed.	
	N/A	Test 1. Eat a small amount of your challenge food. Enter amount here: _____	
	60 minutes	Monitor for a reaction. If there are no symptoms, proceed.	
	N/A	Test 2. Eat a greater amount of your challenge food. Enter amount here: _____	
	60 minutes	Monitor for a reaction. If there are no symptoms, proceed.	
	N/A	Test 3. Eat a greater amount of your challenge food. Enter amount here: _____	
	60 minutes	Monitor for a reaction. If there are no symptoms, proceed.	
	N/A	Test 4. Eat a greater amount of your challenge food. Enter amount here: _____	
	60 minutes	Monitor for a reaction. If there are no symptoms, proceed.	
	N/A	Test 5. Eat a greater amount of your challenge food. Enter amount here: _____	
	60 minutes	Monitor for a reaction. If there are no symptoms, stop for the day.	

Day 2   date: _____

Time	How Long	What to Do	Notes/Symptoms
	All day	Go back to the elimination diet you were on, and simply monitor for a reaction. If there are no symptoms, mark this food as safe for you. You may move on to the next challenge food on day 3 by repeating this process.	

Maintaining: Eating After the Targeted Elimination Diet

The easiest way to do this is to use the food lists in Chapter 17: Maintenance Diet Tools, and cross out any foods that are not allowed for you. Then, using these same sheets, choose only from the safe foods for you. For each meal, choose a vegetable, a protein, and a grain or starch. Add healthy fats to meals and snacks as appropriate (just don't go overboard on calories). You may choose from any of the food lists for your snacks, but it'll probably be easiest to snack on fresh fruit and nuts (if they are safe for you).

1. Go to food lists in maintenance diet tools. Cross out any foods that are not safe for you. Add any favorite safe foods that are missing. This is now your universe of safe foods.

Single Meal

2. For a single meal, choose a food from each group that follows. Putting them together can be as easy as doing a quick Internet search, typing in the foods and the word *recipe*.

Vegetable:

Protein:

Grain or starch:

Meal idea:

Weekly Meals

3. For a week of meals, it is easier to choose a handful of foods from each food list that you'd like to use that week;

Vegetables *(choose three to five different ones, especially dark green and orange)*:

Protein foods *(choose at least three different ones, and try to make at least one a plant protein)*:

Grains or starches *(choose at least two different ones, and try to make at least one a whole grain)*:

4. Mix and match foods so that you always end up with a meal that has a vegetable, a protein, and a grain or starch. Use fresh fish, poultry, and delicate produce (think tender greens, summer squash, or asparagus) at the beginning of the week; use fresh pork or beef midweek through the fifth day; and use heartier vegetables throughout the week (think carrots, onions, potatoes, or winter squash). Plant proteins, such as beans, often last weeks or months, as do frozen versions of fresh meats.

5. Here are my top tips for easy meal planning:

   • Always make enough for next-day leftovers.

   • Choose a few simple foods to have on hand as snacks throughout the week.

   • Don't forget to defrost frozen meats the night before.

   • Include a vegetable or a fruit every time you eat.

   • Don't be fatphobic. Healthy fats are good for you, and add flavor and nutrition to meals.

   • Keep your pantry and freezer stocked with healthy essentials, and you'll always be ready to whip something up.

   • Consider getting a rice cooker or a slow cooker. If you'll be eating a lot of rice, a rice cooker makes it so easy to prepare. A slow cooker can make soups a cinch.

   • Go for seasonal foods. They taste better and will probably be more affordable, too.

   • Don't feel like cooking dinner every night of the week? You'll probably have more than enough food left over to skip making dinner at least one night.

Meal Planner for Targeted Elimination Diet Maintenance Phase

	Breakfast	Lunch	Dinner	Snacks
Day 1				
Day 2				
Day 3				
Day 4				
Day 5				
Day 6				
Day 7				

CHAPTER 14

Catchall Elimination Diet

If you have noticed that you have strong, clear negative reactions to more than five foods on the list of foods allowed on the Targeted Elimination Diet (page 126), you may want to try this more restrictive two-week plan. It's especially useful if you aren't clear how food and your symptoms are connected, as it tends to include only foods that are safe for most people. Then when you begin adding foods back into your diet, it can become clearer what your personal triggers are.

Follow the basic steps of the elimination diet outlined earlier in this book: assess, plan, avoid, challenge, maintain. The following worksheets and charts will help you plan your meals while on the diet, as well as help track any symptoms you may have.

Assess: Food and Symptom Tracker

In the Catchall Elimination Diet, because you may not be sure what role food plays in your symptoms, it's best to stick to distilled or filtered water when washing and cooking food whenever possible. If this is not possible, please make a note of it, as it may be related to your symptoms. Tap water and even non-distilled bottled water may have contaminants that could cause reactions.

Sample Food and Symptom Tracker

Meal	Food/Drink (How Much)	Ingredients	Symptoms
Breakfast Time:	8 oz orange juice 1 Tbsp dry oatmeal with ½ cup hot water	Orange juice, calcium Oatmeal, tap water	Symptoms: Start time: End time: Rating:
AM Snack Time:	23 almonds 1 medium nectarine	Almonds Nectarine	Symptoms: Start time: End time: Rating:
Lunch Time:	1 chicken taco	1 (6-inch) all-natural corn tortilla (corn, water, lime, salt), grilled chicken, coleslaw (cabbage, onion, lime juice, salt, and pepper), salsa (tomatoes, onion, cilantro, lime juice, and salt)	Symptoms: Start time: End time: Rating:
PM Snack Time:	10 oz coffee, 2 oz soy milk, dash cinnamon	Coffee, soy milk (filtered water, whole soybeans), cane sugar, sea salt, carrageenan, natural flavor, calcium carbonate, vitamin A palmitate, vitamin D2, riboflavin (B2), vitamin B12, cinnamon	Symptoms: Start time: End time: Rating:

Meal	Food/Drink (How Much)	Ingredients	Symptoms
Dinner Time:	5 oz baked salmon with lemon and herbs, 1 bunch steamed broccolini, 4 medium roasted red potatoes with rosemary, 10 oz unsweetened ice tea	5 oz salmon, juice of 1 lemon, fresh herbs (dill, parsley), salt; broccolini, water, salt; red potatoes, olive oil, rosemary, salt, pepper; black tea, water, ice	Symptoms: Start time: End time: Rating:
PM Snack Time:	10 oz tart frozen yogurt, plain	Nonfat strained yogurt, nonfat milk, sugar, lemon juice, vanilla extract, salt	Symptoms: Start time: End time: Rating:

Notes: Make a note of anything else that's going on that you think could be affecting how your body reacts, whether it's stress; premenstrual syndrome (PMS); being around animals, gardens, or moldy places; having a cold; or even enjoying a hard workout.

Plan: Prepare Your Pantry for the Catchall Elimination Diet

Pantry Favorites

- Canola oil, safflower oil
- Brown rice
- Rice milk
- Millet
- Rice noodles

- Tapioca
- Rice cereal
- Millet cereal
- Jarred or squeeze pack of pears

- Jarred or squeeze pack of sweet potatoes
- Sea salt
- Distilled water

Freezer Favorites

- Cranberries

- Ground turkey

Fresh Favorites

- Lamb
- Turkey

- Pears
- Cranberries

- Lettuce
- Zucchini

- Summer squash
- Pattypan squash
- Butternut squash
- Acorn squash

- Crookneck squash
- Hubbard squash
- Winter squash
- Spaghetti squash

- Parsnips
- Sweet potatoes
- Yams

Other foods:

- Include fish, fresh or canned, only if turkey or lamb are not tolerated and if fish is tolerated.

Food Guide by Perishability for the Catchall Elimination Diet

High Perishability use up in 1 to 2 days	Medium Perishability use up in 3 to 4 days	Low Perishability use up anytime in the week	Very Low Perishability lasts a week or longer
Fish (flounder, salmon, tuna)	Lamb Turkey	Frozen lamb or turkey	Canned fish
	Lettuce Pattypan squash Summer squash Zucchini	Acorn squash Butternut squash Parsnips Spaghetti squash Sweet potatoes Winter squash Yams	Jarred or frozen pure versions of OK vegetables Millet (.e.g., millet cereal, millet) Rice (e.g., rice cereal, rice milk, rice noodles, rice) Tapioca
Fresh juice from OK fruits and vegetables (fresh pear juice, homemade cranberry juice)		Cranberries Pears	Jarred or frozen pure versions of OK fruits and pear juice
Tapioca pudding (made with OK ingredients) Rice pudding (made with OK ingredients)			Canola and safflower oil Distilled water Sea salt

Eliminate: Begin Your Catchall Elimination Diet

This is a two-week plan. One week of meals has been provided, and can be repeated for the second week. As this is a restrictive diet that requires many changes from the regular diet, there may be comfort in having some consistency from week to week.

Creating meal plans can be challenging even without food restrictions, but the process is the same. You start with a set of foods and mix and match to create meals and snacks, being sure to use up more perishable foods earlier in the week. Here, I've created weekly meal plans to take some of the work out of your elimination diet. The week starts on Saturday, when you are more likely to have time to cook.

I have provided meal plans for the short-term elimination diet (very few foods) as well as the lifestyle elimination diet (free of all major allergens and processed foods).

Week 1 Meal Plan for the Catchall Elimination Diet

	Breakfast	Lunch/Dinner	Lunch/Dinner	Snacks
Monday	Rice crackers with homemade cranberry jam	Tuna with mashed parsnips and pattypan squash meal leftovers	Turkey meatballs over spaghetti squash	Fresh pear slices
Tuesday	Brown rice porridge with chopped pears and cranberries	Turkey meatball and spaghetti squash meal leftovers	Broiled lamb over brown rice with sautéed zucchini rounds	Turkey meatballs
Wednesday	Millet porridge with chopped cranberries	Millet, tuna, and lettuce salad with canned tuna	Lamb with brown rice and zucchini meal leftovers	Baked pear with cranberry jam
Thursday	Rice crackers with mashed yam spread and slices of pears	Zucchini-tapioca soup	Millet-salmon cakes over bed of lettuce	Popped millet (similar to popcorn)
Friday	Pear-millet breakfast tart	Millet-salmon cakes over bed of lettuce leftovers	Zucchini and millet risotto with millet-yam-cranberry-pear tart	Small piece of millet-yam-cranberry-pear tart
Saturday	Brown rice porridge topped with chopped zucchini	Butternut squash, acorn squash, and pear soup	Flounder with brown rice and sautéed summer squash	Baked baby jewel yams, perfect for individual snacks
Sunday	Butternut squash, acorn squash, and pear soup	Brown rice porridge topped with chopped zucchini	Tuna steak with a side of mashed parsnips and pattypan squash	Baked baby jewel yams, perfect for individual snacks

Week 1 Grocery List

Pantry (you may already have)

  • Brown rice, millet, tapioca

  • Rice crackers

Perishable (buy fresh)

  • *Fruit:* Cranberries, pears

  • *Vegetable:* Acorn squash, baby jewel yams, butternut squash, lettuce, parsnips, pattypan squash, spaghetti squash, summer squash, yams, zucchini

  • *Meat:* Ground turkey, lamb

  • *Fish (fresh or canned, only if tolerated):* Tuna, salmon, flounder

Recipes for the Catchall Elimination Diet

Brown Rice Porridge Topped with Chopped Zucchini

On the Catchall Elimination Diet, your meals are defined by simplicity.
This hearty warm breakfast is simple and satisfying.

1 cup brown rice   1 zucchini, washed and chopped

1 Tbsp canola oil

1. If you have a rice cooker, prepare brown rice in advance. (Rice porridge is also a great way to use leftover rice.) If using already cooked rice, combine with six additional cups of water in a large pot, bring to a boil, and then reduce heat to a simmer. Let simmer until it reaches a consistency you like. It may be an hour for a more watery porridge, and 1.5–2 hours for a thicker porridge. (If using uncooked rice, combine 1 cup rice and 8 cups of water, bring to boil, and then simmer to desired consistency.)

2. Add canola oil to a sauté pan, and sauté zucchini for just a few minutes until just cooked. Add salt to season if desired.

3. Top porridge with zucchini and enjoy.

4. Porridge can be reheated the next day in the microwave or on the stove top. (Add more water if it's become thicker than you like.)

Butternut Squash, Acorn Squash, and Pear Soup

You can mix and match for this soup using any allowed squash, but as
with all catchall recipes, this will be a simple preparation.

1 butternut squash, halved, seeded   1 Tbsp oil

1 acorn squash, halved, seeded   Salt, to taste

2 pears, chopped

1. Preheat oven to 350 degrees F.

2. Place butternut squash and acorn squash, cut side down, on a baking dish, and roast for about 45–60 minutes. The squash should be tender. For a shortcut, place squash, cut side down, on a microwave-safe plate, and cook on high for 5 minutes. Check for tenderness and, if needed, heat for another couple of minutes before checking again. Either way, when it's cool enough to touch, scoop out the insides and place in a large pot with four cups of water.

3. Heat large pot of squash-and-water mixture on medium-high heat until it comes to a boil. Reduce to a simmer.

4. Meanwhile, sauté chopped pears in oil until softened, and then add to large pot.

5. Simmer until soup reaches desired thickness. Season with salt to taste.

6. Alternatively, combine the squash and the pears in a blender for a smoother soup. The preceding simpler process makes a more rustic soup.

Turkey Meatballs Over Spaghetti Squash

1 spaghetti squash	1 cup brown rice, cooked
Oil, to taste	2 Tbsp oil
Salt, to taste	1 tsp salt
1 lb ground turkey	½ cup fresh cranberries (optional)

1. Preheat oven to 350 degrees F.

2. Pierce spaghetti squash with a fork or sharp knife to create "vents," so that it doesn't explode everywhere.

3. Place whole spaghetti squash on baking pan, and bake for about an hour (or bake in microwave on high for 10–15 minutes, stopping once in the middle, and waiting a good 10 minutes afterward to let it cool down a little).

4. While the spaghetti squash is baking, combine ground turkey, cooked rice, the 2 Tbsp oil, and salt until it forms a dough of sorts. Roll into 24 mini-meatballs, and place evenly on a baking sheet.

5. Bake for 20 minutes and then check for doneness. If done, remove from oven. If not, let bake an additional 5–10 minutes before checking again. Turkey must be cooked to 165 degrees F to be safe. You can add the turkey meatballs right into the same oven as the spaghetti squash to save on time.

6. Once the spaghetti squash is cool enough to handle, carefully cut it open lengthwise, being aware of hot steam. Oven mitts may help. Remove the seeds. Then use a fork to scrape out the rest of the squash into a large bowl. It should come out in strings resembling strands of spaghetti. Add oil and salt to taste and toss.

7. When everything is cooked thoroughly, portion out a serving of spaghetti squash and top with turkey meatballs.

8. For a tart twist, top this dish with fresh cranberries, chopped in a food processor.

Pear-Millet Breakfast Tart

1 cup dry millet	Mashed sweet potatoes (optional)
3 cups water	Oil, to taste
1 Tbsp oil	Salt, to taste
1 tsp salt	Chopped fresh cranberries (optional)
3 pears	

1. Preheat oven to 350 degrees F.

2. Toast millet in a skillet over medium heat for a few minutes until it starts to smell nutty.

3. In a medium pot, combine toasted millet and water, bring to a boil, and then reduce heat to a simmer. Add the 1 Tbsp oil and 1 tsp salt, and cover to let simmer for about 15 minutes.

4. Remove from heat and let rest (it's finishing cooking) for another 10-15 minutes. It'll be a little sticky.

5. Slice pears in thin, flat slices.

6. Spread cooked millet in a thin layer on the bottom of a baking pan. If you have leftover mashed sweet potatoes, add a layer of this to the dish. Then top with slices of pear. Drizzle with oil, sprinkle with salt, and then place in oven to bake for another 5-10 minutes, until the millet has thickened and looks more like a crust.

7. Enjoy warm! Optional: Try topping the warm dish with chopped fresh cranberries for a tart accent.

Single-ingredient-based snacks and recipes

The catchall diet is all about simplicity. That's why I'm including a number of single-ingredient recipe ideas to help add some variety to a diet with a limited number of foods. And OK, some of the ideas include 2–3 ingredients.

Pears

- Whole pears
- Pear smoothie with blended pears and ice
- Broiled pears (with or without oil and sprinkle of salt)
- Dried pear rings
- Pear puree Popsicles

Butternut squash

- Butternut squash chips baked with oil and salt
- Millet
- Popped millet (Heat millet in a skillet until it smells nutty. Stir and then wait. In 3–5 minutes, the millet should start popping just like stove-top popcorn does. Just remove it from the heat when it's all popped, so that it doesn't overcook.)

Tapioca

- Tapioca "pudding" made with rice milk

Sweet potatoes

- Baked sweet potatoes

- Mashed sweet potatoes

- Sweet potato baked slices

Parsnips

- Mashed parsnips

Rice

- Rice cakes

- Rice cereal

- Rice milk (If you can't find any with only allowed ingredients, you can make your own with cooked rice and water at a 1:4 ratio, simmer until combined, and then pop the mixture into a blender. The final step is straining it through a fine mesh strainer or cheesecloth.)

Squash (any)

- Simple soups made with pureed squash, water, and allowed seasonings

Challenge: Identifying Your Challenge Foods

For the Catchall Elimination Diet, you will be looking into your own past diet for suspicious foods. Go through your initial food and symptom tracker, and circle any food that shows up more than twice a week. Use the space that follows to write down some of the more commonly eaten foods by category, starting with the foods that you ate the most of, the most often.

Vegetables:

Fruit:

Animal protein:

Plant protein:

Grains:

Oils or fats:

Processed snacks:

Other:

Open Food Challenge Worksheet

Challenge food: _____

How much would you normally consume in a day? _____

Divide by 4: _X_

- Test 1 amount: _1/2X_

- Test 2 amount: _X_

- Test 3 amount: _2X_

- Test 4 amount: _4X_

- Test 5 amount: _8X_

For example, if you are challenging with milk, and you normally drink an 8-oz glass of milk a day, you would fill in the blanks like this:

Challenge Food: _milk_

How much would you normally consume in a day? _8 oz_

- Divide by 4: _2 oz_

- Test 1 amount: _1 oz_

- Test 2 amount: _2 oz_

- Test 3 amount: _4 oz_

- Test 4 amount: _8 oz_

- Test 5 amount: _16 oz_

As soon as you react to a food, make a note of it and stop the food challenge. Then follow directions for outcome 2, which follows.

At the end of the challenge, please check one of these boxes:

[   ] Outcome 1: This food is safe for me!

This is great news. However, still keep this food out of the diet for the rest of the challenge phase to keep the results clear.

[   ] Outcome 2: This food caused symptoms.

If this is the case, go back to the elimination diet for as long as it takes for symptoms to resolve, whether that's one day or seven (or more). Once symptoms have cleared up, wait an additional two days before going on to the next challenge.

Open Food Challenge Worksheet

Day 1

date: _____

Time	How Long	What to Do	Notes/Symptoms
	2 minutes	Put food on lower lip.	
	30 minutes	Monitor for a reaction. If there are no symptoms, proceed.	
	N/A	Test 1. Eat a small amount of your challenge food Enter amount here: _____	
	60 minutes	Monitor for a reaction. If there are no symptoms, proceed.	
	N/A	Test 2. Eat a greater amount of your challenge food. Enter amount here: _____	
	60 minutes	Monitor for a reaction. If there are no symptoms, proceed.	
	N/A	Test 3. Eat a greater amount of your challenge food. Enter amount here: _____	
	60 minutes	Monitor for a reaction. If there are no symptoms, proceed.	
	N/A	Test 4. Eat a greater amount of your challenge food. Enter amount here: _____	
	60 minutes	Monitor for a reaction. If there are no symptoms, proceed.	
	N/A	Test 5. Eat a greater amount of your challenge food. Enter amount here: _____	
	60 minutes	Monitor for a reaction. If there are no symptoms, stop for the day.	

Day 2

date: _____

Time	How Long	What to Do	Notes/Symptoms
	All day	Go back to the elimination diet you were on, and simply monitor for a reaction.	
		If there are no symptoms, mark this food as safe for you. You may move on to the next challenge food on day 3 by repeating this process.	

Maintaining: Eating After the Catchall Elimination Diet

The easiest way to do this is to use the food lists in Chapter 17: Maintenance Diet Tools, and cross out any foods that are not allowed for you. Then, using these same sheets, choose only from the safe foods for you. For each meal, choose a vegetable, a protein, and a grain or starch. Add healthy fats to meals and snacks as appropriate (just don't go overboard on calories). You may choose from any of the food lists for your snacks, but it'll probably be easiest to snack on fresh fruit and nuts (if they are safe for you).

Chapter 15

Tip Sheets for Avoiding Common Allergens

Reading Food Labels 101

When you look at a food label, you will be focusing first and foremost on the ingredients statement to make sure that all the ingredients in a given food are safe for you. Secondarily, it's great to look at the nutrition to make sure the food has something of value, such as being a good source of fiber, protein, vitamins, calcium, or other minerals, and that it doesn't have an excessive amount of saturated fat, sodium, or sugar.

I'm trying to avoid the eight major allergens. What should I look for on the food label?

You're in luck. The FDA requires that packaged foods that contain any of the eight major allergens (i.e., milk, eggs, wheat, peanuts, soy, tree nuts, fish, and shellfish) must label them.

The law requires that food labels identify the food source names of all major food allergens used to make the food. This requirement is met if the common or usual name of an ingredient (e.g., buttermilk) that is a major food allergen already identifies that allergen's food source name (i.e., milk). Otherwise, the allergen's food source name must be declared at least once on the food label in one of two ways:

1. In parentheses following the name of the ingredient. Examples: "lecithin (soy)," "flour (wheat)," and "whey (milk)."

2. Immediately after or next to the list of ingredients in a "contains" statement. Example: "Contains wheat, milk, and soy."

Some labels say, "Contains [allergen X]," and some say, "May contain [allergen X]." What's the difference?

If it says "Contains milk," for example, this means the product definitely contains a milk ingredient. But the "May contain" statement is voluntary. For example, if a rice cereal was processed on the same production line as a wheat cereal, then wheat wouldn't show up in the ingredients. But there's a pretty strong chance for cross-contact, so the manufacturer might label its product with the statement, "May contain wheat." Because it's voluntary, it's a good idea to follow up with a manufacturer directly if you are worried about cross-contact.

Tips for Reading Food Labels

1. Check before you buy. Ingredients can and do change over time, so it's important to check the label every time.

2. Become familiar with the less obvious key words that are associated with the food you are avoiding (e.g., if you're avoiding milk, know that "lacto," "casein," and "whey" often indicate that milk is present).

3. Be aware that vague terms, such as "spices," or "natural flavors," don't always give you enough information, and you'll want to contact the manufacturer directly to find out if it's safe for you.

4. Food isn't the only thing that contains food-type ingredients. Check the ingredients on toiletries (e.g., lotions), cosmetics (e.g., lipstick), and household cleaners you come into contact with (e.g., soaps).

Free Resource to Help You Avoid the Eight Major Allergens

For tips on how to read a label to avoid the eight major allergens, check out this resource from Food Allergy Research and Education (FARE): http://www.foodallergy.org/document.doc?id=133

The tip sheets in Chapter 16 on how to avoid certain foods provide more detailed information about specific foods. Tip sheets are included on how to avoid milk, eggs, wheat, peanuts, soy, tree nuts, fish, and shellfish, as well as sulfites, tartrazine, benzoates, MSG, nickel, and corn.

Strategies for Life Situations

At Home

If it's easy, just get the offending food out of your kitchen. Clean out your pantry, refrigerator, and freezer. This is no problem if you live by yourself. When you have a roommate, spouse, or children to consider, you'll have to see how they feel about it. If it's not ideal for them, keep offending foods separate from your foods. And it's a good idea to keep it on lower shelves, so that it's less likely to make contact with other foods. Clean up with soap and water after a meal. Wash hands before and after eating. Use separate cooking utensils and plates. Thoroughly clean counters, cutting boards, knives, and so on, in between prepping foods. A lot of these are good food safety practices anyway.

Dining Out

- Ask for recommendations from people who have food sensitivities. This is when it's great to be part of a regional support group. There may even be mentions of a restaurant's policy in Yelp reviews. Many restaurants are now much more aware of sensitivities and gluten-free eating.

- If it's a group dinner, offer to do the research to find a few good options for the group. You can ensure that they all meet your needs, while offering up a few different selections for your friends. It's not your fault you have food sensitivities, but it's not everyone else's either. The classy thing to do is to offer up a solution.

- Beware of desserts unless the pastry chef works on-site and you can get answers to your questions. Many restaurants outsource their desserts, so they may not have any control over cross-contact. This tip really goes for any food that looks as though it's been prepped elsewhere.

- Order simple foods.

- Stay away from buffets. Cross-contact is all but inevitable.

- Avoid restaurants that feature your trigger foods. For example, if fish bothers you, don't pick a seafood restaurant. If peanuts trouble you, stay away from Thai restaurants.

- Call ahead and speak to a manager about your food sensitivities. You'll get a good idea whether they are cautious about sensitivities. If you decide to give the restaurant a try, ask your server a lot of questions.

- Bring your own safe foods, just in case. It's clearly not ideal, but it's better than nothing. If the main reason is to get together with others, let that be the highlight of your evening rather than the food.

Traveling

Wanderlust. It's practically baked into human DNA. For air travel, check the airline's snack offerings online. When you book your flight, if there's an area for special meal request notes, you can include the foods you are sensitive to. Given the way many airlines operate these days, the most you may have to do is decline their complimentary snack offering and bring your own meal (because you would have to pay for a meal anyway). International flights are more challenging. You'll have to get really good at communicating your food sensitivity to flight attendants. Check out your seat and make sure there are no food remnants, such as crumbs, that may cause you discomfort. And maybe bring hand sanitizer or sanitation wipes to wipe down surfaces. Just try to do it without much fuss. You are doing something to keep yourself healthy. It's OK to do this, but it doesn't define you. You can politely tell those sitting next to you. But they should be free to eat whatever they want. Just be cautious. Do some research into restaurants at your destination. Bring nonperishable, practical snacks that you know are safe for you, such as nutrition bars. Maybe look up key words in the language of the foreign country if you are doing international travel. For example, if you do not drink cow's milk, learn the words for soy milk and almond milk in other languages, so you can request it with coffee, tea, or breakfast. Bring your own food.

Cross-Contact 101

Cross-contact occurs when a trigger food comes into contact with otherwise safe food. It can be managed by taking precautions when storing foods and by good cleaning practices. It's a good idea to keep a separate area to store and prepare food and to store kitchen tools, including cutting boards, utensils, pots and pans, plates, and so on. Good cleaning technique can safely remove all the trigger food from a surface, so be sure to wash the surfaces with soap and water. Wiping isn't enough.

For packaged foods, cross-contact can happen during the manufacturing and processing of the food. Manufacturing plants seldom produce only one food, which means that the building and the production lines are shared by multiple foods. If one of the foods is a trigger food for you, there is the possibility of an unsafe cross-contact. If you are concerned, get in touch with the manufacturer; most major manufacturers are ready to answer these questions for customers.

At delis and grocery stores, cross-contact can happen if the same tools are used to touch different foods. For example, a scooping spoon, knives, or a deli slicer that is used for both meat and cheese can mean that an unsafe cross-contact occurs. Bulk bins are another example. Even an invisible trace of food on a spoon or spatula can cause an allergic reaction.

At restaurants and at home, if the same cooking utensils are used for safe and unsafe foods, an unsafe cross-contact can occur. Trigger foods can come into contact with safe foods from hands as well, so it's important to wash hands and utensils in between preparing different foods. For example, when a knife that has been used to spread peanut butter is only wiped clean before being used to spread jelly, an unsafe cross-contact can occur.

At breakfast, the grill might be used to scramble eggs and cook French toast, so the grill would contain egg, milk, and wheat proteins. At lunch, the grill might be used to cook meats. These items may not contain egg, milk, or wheat proteins, but if the grill was not properly cleaned before lunch, the allergens would still be present.

Alternative Foods for Key Nutrients

The eight classes of food that are responsible for 90 percent of the allergenic reactions are milk, eggs, wheat, peanuts, soy, tree nuts, fish, and shellfish. In their pure form, these are also foods that provide important nutrients for good health. When a food needs to be avoided because of food sensitivities, it's important to understand what key nutrients to make up for. At least thirty-four nutrients are needed to keep the body healthy. Thankfully, these important nutrients come from many different foods, so a well-balanced and varied diet should provide ample opportunity for a nutritionally complete diet. However, certain nutrients are "shortfall nutrients" in the United States. That is to say, most Americans aren't getting enough of certain nutrients. These are vitamin D, calcium, potassium, and fiber.

Following is an at-a-glance guide to which of the major allergens are important sources of these important nutrients, along with alternative sources. If you're sensitive to only one food type, then you may be able to eat the other major potential allergens just fine. In case you need to avoid more than one major allergen, the eight major allergens are highlighted at each place where one of the eight is discussed.

Alternative Nutritional Sources

Food	Shortfall Nutrient	Alternative Sources
Milk	Calcium	Ready-to-eat cereal (fortified), orange juice (fortified), tofu (made with calcium sulfate), sardines, soy milk (fortified), rice milk (fortified)
Milk (fortified)	Vitamin D	Salmon, rockfish, tuna, sardines, soy milk (fortified), flounder, sole, rice milk (fortified), herring, pork, orange juice (fortified), shiitake mushrooms
Milk	Potassium	Potatoes, prune juice, carrot juice, tomato paste, cooked beet greens, canned white beans, canned tomato juice, tomato puree, sweet potatoes, clams, orange juice, halibut, soybeans, tuna, lima beans, rockfish, Pacific cod, bananas, spinach, tomato sauce, dried peaches, prunes, rainbow trout, dried apricots, pinto beans, pork loin, lentils, plantains, kidney beans, coffee
Eggs	Vitamin D	Salmon, rockfish, tuna, sardines, soy milk (fortified), flounder, sole, rice milk (fortified), herring, pork, orange juice (fortified), shiitake mushrooms, milk (fortified)
Wheat	Fiber	Beans and legumes (navy beans, split peas, lentils, pinto beans, black beans, chickpeas, and so on), pistachios, almonds, apples, pears, bananas, green peas, sweet potatoes, potatoes, edamame, spinach, oranges, winter squash, parsnips, collard greens, broccoli, okra, turnip greens
Soy	Fiber (soybeans)	Beans and legumes (navy beans, split peas, lentils, pinto beans, black beans, chickpeas, and so on, but not soybeans), pistachios, almonds, apples, pears, bananas, green peas, sweet potatoes, potatoes, spinach, oranges, winter squash, parsnips, collard greens, broccoli, okra, turnip greens, whole grains (e.g., wheat bran, rye wafers, bulgur, quinoa, popcorn, and so on)
Soy	Potassium	Potatoes, prune juice, carrot juice, tomato paste, cooked beet greens, canned white beans, canned tomato juice, tomato puree, sweet potatoes, clams, orange juice, halibut, tuna, lima beans, rockfish, Pacific cod, bananas, spinach, tomato sauce, dried peaches, prunes, rainbow trout, dried apricots, pinto beans, pork loin, lentils, plantains, kidney beans, coffee
Soy (fortified)	Vitamin D (fortified)	Salmon, rockfish, tuna, sardines, flounder, sole, rice milk (fortified), herring, pork, orange juice (fortified), shiitake mushrooms, milk (fortified), eggs
Soy (fortified)	Calcium	Ready-to-eat cereal (fortified), orange juice (fortified), sardines, rice milk (fortified), milk, yogurt, cheese
Peanuts	N/A	N/A
Tree nuts	Fiber	Beans and legumes (navy beans, split peas, lentils, pinto beans, black beans, chickpeas, soybeans, and so on), apples, pears, bananas, green peas, sweet potatoes, potatoes, spinach, orange, winter squash, parsnips, collard greens, broccoli, okra, turnip greens, whole grains (e.g., wheat bran, rye wafers, bulgur, quinoa, popcorn, and so on)
Fish	Vitamin D	Soy milk (fortified), rice milk (fortified), pork, orange juice (fortified), shiitake mushrooms, milk (fortified), eggs
Fish	Potassium	Potatoes, prune juice, carrot juice, tomato paste, cooked beet greens, canned white beans, canned tomato juice, tomato puree, sweet potatoes, orange juice, soybeans, lima beans, bananas, spinach, tomato sauce, dried peaches, prunes, dried apricots, pinto beans, pork loin, lentils, plantains, kidney beans, coffee
Shellfish	Vitamin D	Salmon, rockfish, tuna, sardines, soy milk (fortified), flounder, sole, rice milk (fortified), herring, pork, orange juice (fortified), shiitake mushrooms, milk (fortified)

Substitutions

Food	Use	Substitute
Milk	Hot cereal, cold cereal, coffee, tea, beverage	Rice milk, oat milk, almond milk, almond-coconut milk
Milk	Calcium	Dark leafy greens, such as bok choy, broccoli, collard greens, kale
Milk	Cream, sour cream, yogurts, cheeses, frozen desserts	Almond milk, soy milk, rice milk
Eggs	Protein	Poultry, meat, plant proteins (legumes, nuts)
Eggs	Breakfast	Egg-free egg substitutes
Eggs	Mayonnaise	Vegan mayonnaise
Wheat	Grain, starch, fiber	Rice, millet, quinoa, corn, sweet potatoes, potatoes, winter squash, gluten-free pastas, breads, crackers, and so on
Wheat	Beer	Gluten-free beer
Peanuts	Baking, cooking	Tree nuts, almond butter, pumpkin seed butter, soy butter
Peanuts	Snacks	Baked chickpeas, popped millet, tree nuts, water chestnuts, popcorn, pumpkin seeds, sunflower seeds
Tree nuts	Baking, cooking	Alternative tree nuts, peanuts
Tree nuts	Snacks	Alternative tree nuts, baked chickpeas, popped millet, tree nuts, water chestnuts, popcorn, pumpkin seeds, sunflower seeds
Tree nuts and peanuts	Healthy fats	Avocados, fatty fish, alternative tree nuts
Soy	Plant protein	Legumes and beans, including black beans, pinto beans, black-eyed peas, chickpeas, lentils, split peas, white beans, navy beans, and so on
Soy	Soy sauce	Coconut-based amino acids (at natural food stores)
Fish	Protein	Poultry, meat, plant proteins (legumes, nuts)
Fish	Omega-3s	Walnuts, flax
Shellfish	Protein	Poultry, meat, plant proteins (legumes, nuts)

CHAPTER 16

Tip Sheets for Avoiding Common Trigger Foods

How to Avoid Sulfites

There's a good chance you'll find sulfites in fruit products (juice, pulp, syrup, salad, spreads, candied fruit, such as cherries and fruit peels, fruity ice cream, fruit fillings, canned or dehydrated fruit), vegetable products (juice, canned or dehydrated vegetables, dried ginger root), instant soup or mashed potatoes, dried fruit (e.g., dried bananas, apricots, and coconut), jams, jellies, and marmalades, pickles and relish, beer and wine (including the nonalcoholic versions), cider, and cider vinegar, canned crabmeat, preserved egg yolk, powdered garlic, concentrated pineapple juice, caramel coloring, bleached cod, bleached white sugar, certain frozen foods (potatoes, sliced mushrooms, sliced apples, shrimp, prawn, lobster), any pudding with gelatin, sausage, soft drinks, pectin, dextrose, molasses, tomato products (paste, pulp, ketchup, puree), grapes. There are test strips on the market that can be used to check whether sulfites are in food, but they are often unreliable and so not recommended.

Labeling Smarts

Sulfites in the ingredients may be listed as sodium sulfite, sulfur dioxide, sodium bisulfite, potassium bisulfate, sodium metabisulfite, potassium metabisulfite, sulfurous acid. According to the FDA, if sulfites can be detected at or over 10 ppm (parts per million), then they have to be listed in the ingredients statement, whether the sulfites are natural or added. Also, any sulfites added as a preservative must be labeled, even if the sulfites are below the 10 ppm level.

The FDA banned the use of sulfites on fresh fruits and vegetables in 1986, except for fresh grapes and sliced potatoes. The FDA also keeps sulfites out of enriched flours and grains because they provide an essential B vitamin called thiamine, which is destroyed by sulfites. Read all product labels carefully before purchasing and consuming any item. Ingredients in packaged food products may change without warning, so check ingredient statements carefully every time you shop. If you have questions, call the manufacturer.

What You Can Eat

- Fruits and vegetables: All whole, uncut, and fresh fruits and vegetables, except grapes or potatoes
- Protein: Fresh poultry and meat, fin fish (but not shellfish), processed meats that are labeled as sulfite-free, beans and legumes, nuts, seeds
- Dairy: Milk, buttermilk, cream, sour cream, yogurt, cheese, cottage and ricotta cheese, butter
- Grains: Whole-grain flours, plain pasta, breakfast cereal without dried fruit or coconut
- Oils: Nuts, seeds, vegetable oil
- Packaged foods: Any foods that do not have sulfites listed in ingredients or are labeled as sulfite-free
- Beverages: Water, coffee, rice milk, almond milk, soy milk

Foods and Ingredients to Avoid

- Alcoholic and nonalcoholic beer and cider
- Bottled lemon and lime juices and concentrates
- Canned and frozen fruits and vegetables
- Cereal, cornmeal, cornstarch, crackers, and muesli
- Condiments, for example coleslaw dressing, horseradish, ketchup, mustard, pickles, relish, and sauerkraut
- Dehydrated, mashed, peeled, and precut potatoes and frozen French fries
- Dried fruits and vegetables, such as apricots, coconut, and raisins; sweet potatoes
- Dried herbs, spices, and teas
- Fresh grapes
- Fruit fillings and syrups, gelatin, jams, jellies, preserves, marmalade, molasses and pectin
- Fruit and vegetable juices
- Glazed and glacéed fruits, for example maraschino cherries

- Starches, for example cornstarch, potato starch

- Sugar syrups, for example glucose, glucose solids, syrup dextrose, corn syrup, table syrup

- Tomato pastes, pulps, and purees

- Vinegar and wine vinegar

- Wine

Other Possible Sources of Sulfites

- Baked goods, especially those with dried fruits

- Deli meats, hot dogs, and sausages

- Dressings, gravies, guacamole, sauces, soups, and soup mixes

- Fish, crustaceans, and shellfish

- Granola bars, especially those with dried fruit

- Noodle and rice mixes

- Snack foods, for example raisins, fruit salad

- Soy products

Nonfood Sources of Sulfites

Many medications contain sulfites, so be sure to talk to your pharmacist about your sulfites sensitivity. It's important to ask every time, because medication formulations change.

Plastic bags and other packaging might be sanitized with sulfites. It's possible to be exposed to sulfites when opening a bag that has been sanitized this way; be especially cautious when opening up a bag of dried fruit, as both are potential ways to expose yourself to sulfites. These sulfites don't need to be in the ingredients statement but could still be a concern if you're sensitive.

How to Avoid Tartrazine

You have so many options for what to eat when you have a tartrazine sensitivity. Anything in its whole, natural state is fine, as is anything that is USDA certified as organic. That's because whole foods and organic foods do not contain artificial colors.

What You Can Eat

- Fruits and vegetables: all fresh; for frozen, canned, or jarred, check the label

- Protein: fresh fish, poultry, and meat

- Dairy or calcium: plain milk, butter, check labels on other dairy foods for tartrazine, FD&C Yellow #5, Yellow No. 5, or Yellow 5

- Grains: all plain grains, such as brown rice, wild rice, whole wheat pasta; for other than plain grains and mixes, check the ingredients label

- Oils (most oils will be OK as additives are uncommon; to confirm, simply look at the ingredients, which should be simple, such as canola oil, extra virgin olive oil, and so on)

- Beverages: water, tea, coffee, 100 percent fruit or vegetable juice

- Other: there may be versions of the foods most likely to contain tartrazine that are specially made without it; check food labels to be sure, so you don't have to miss out on a favorite food if there is a tartrazine-free alternative

Labeling Smarts

Tartrazine will most likely show up in an ingredients statement simply as Yellow No. 5, though it may also be referenced as Yellow 5 or FD&C Yellow #5. This artificial food coloring is classified as an FDA-certified color additive, and anything that falls into that category must be called out by name in the ingredients statement. This means that if you see "artificial colors" listed in the ingredients without specifics, the food doesn't contain Yellow 5.

Read all product labels carefully before purchasing and consuming any item. Ingredients in packaged food products may change without warning, so check ingredient statements carefully every time you shop. If you have questions, call the manufacturer.

Foods and Ingredients to Avoid

The following foods may have tartrazine (FD&C Yellow #5) in them, though not all of them do. Some manufacturers create their products without artificial colors. Be sure to take a close look at the ingredients statement.

- Aproten (low-protein pasta products)

- Bottled sauces

- Butterscotch chips

- Cake mixes

- Cake mixes, commercial pies

- Candy

- Certain breakfast cereals
- Certain candy coatings
- Certain ice creams and sherbets
- Certain instant and regular puddings
- Chewing gum
- Chocolate chips
- Colored marshmallows
- Colored sodas
- Commercial frostings
- Commercial gingerbread
- Dried or canned soup
- Flavored carbonated beverages
- Flavored drink mixes
- Flavored yogurts and milks

- Fruit punch
- Gelatin
- Hard candies
- Ice cream
- Instant pudding
- Jams
- Jellies
- Mustard
- Pickles
- Ready-to-eat canned puddings
- Refrigerated rolls and quick breads
- Salad dressing, store-bought
- Smoked fish

How to Avoid Benzoates

Benzoates are chemicals that are used as food additives, though some are found naturally in foods.

What You Can Eat

- Fruits and vegetables: apples, persimmon, grapes, kiwifruit, onion, cauliflower, celery, lettuce, cabbage, potatoes, broccoli

- Protein: fresh fish, poultry, and meat

- Oils: oils without hydrolyzed lecithin in ingredients—olive oil, most vegetable oils (check labels)

- Beverages: water, plain coffee, wine

Labeling Smarts

On a food label, benzoates can show up as benzoic acid, sodium benzoate, potassium benzoate, calcium benzoate, and a few other names, which you'll be able to spot because they end in "benzoate."

Read all product labels carefully before purchasing and consuming any item. Ingredients in packaged food products may change without warning, so check ingredient statements carefully every time you shop. If you have questions, call the manufacturer.

Foods and Ingredients to Avoid

Natural sources higher in benzoates

- Apricots
- Avocados
- Cinnamon
- Cherries
- Clove
- Cranberries
- Honey
- Nectarine
- Nutmeg
- Oranges
- Papayas
- Peaches
- Pimento
- Plums
- Prunes
- Pumpkin
- Raspberries
- Red bean
- Soy sauce
- Soybean
- Spinach
- Strawberries
- Thyme
- Tea

May want to avoid these categories

- Berries
- Citrus fruit
- Stone fruit

Foods lower in benzoates

- Almond
- Baked goods
- Banana
- Barbecue sauce
- Barley
- Bay leaf
- Beer
- Black pepper
- Bleached flours
- Candies
- Candy
- Carrots

- Cashew
- Caviar
- Celery seed
- Chinese cabbage
- Chocolate
- Clove
- Cod
- Coffee and chicory essence
- Concentrated fruit juice
- Cooked or packaged beets
- Coriander
- Corn
- Cumin
- Dessert sauces
- Dill pickles
- Fig
- Flavored coffee
- Flavored syrups
- Flavorings for drinks
- Food colorings
- Foods containing hydrolyzed lecithin, such as margarine
- Frozen desserts
- Fruit juice
- Fruit pie fillings
- Fruit pulp or puree
- Garlic

- Gum
- Hazelnut
- Ice cream
- Icing
- Jam
- Jellies
- Kumquat
- Lemon
- Lime
- Mandarin orange
- Margarine
- Marinated fish
- Mustard seed
- Nutmeg
- Oyster sauce
- Paprika
- Pickles
- Pie
- Pimento
- Pineapple
- Pistachio
- Pomegranate
- Prawns
- Quince
- Radish
- Rice
- Salad dressing

- Sesame seed
- Soft drinks
- Soy sauce
- Table olives
- Taco sauce
- Tomato
- Tomato ketchup

- Walnut
- Watermelon
- Wheat
- White pepper
- Worcestershire sauce
- Yogurt

How to Avoid MSG

Hydrolyzed plant protein results in MSG, so keep an eye out for these terms in the ingredients statement: hydrolyzed plant protein, hydrolyzed vegetable protein, hydrolyzed soy protein, autolyzed yeast extract, hydrolyzed yeast, yeast extract, soy extract, protein isolate. MSG is also naturally found in tomatoes and cheese. The FDA doesn't allow foods with these ingredients to have "No MSG" or "No added MSG" claims, even if the source of MSG is natural. The FDA also states that MSG cannot be listed as "spices and flavoring."

Foods and Ingredients to Avoid

- Accent
- Ajinomoto
- Cheeses
- Chinese seasoning
- Flavorings
- Glutacyl
- Glutavene
- Gourmet powder
- HPP
- HVP
- Kombu extract
- Mei-jing

- Monoammonium glutamate
- Monopotassium glutamate
- Mushrooms
- Natural flavoring
- RL-50
- Soy sauce
- Subu
- Tomatoes
- Vetsin
- Wei-jing
- Zest

Processed Foods that Might Contain MSG

- Bottled and canned sauces
- Canned meats
- Canned soups
- Cookies and crackers
- Croutons
- Cured meats
- Diet foods
- Dry soup mixes
- Freeze-dried foods
- Frozen foods
- Gravy
- Mayonnaise
- Potato chips
- Prepared dinners and side dishes
- Prepared salads
- Prepared snacks
- Salad dressings
- Seasoning mixes
- Smoked meats and sausages

How to Avoid Nickel

Nickel is everywhere. It's part of the Earth's crust, so it's in the very soil that grows all of our food. Plants tend to have more nickel than meat does. The amount of nickel in food varies depending on the nickel content of the soil (plants really are what they eat, aka the soil), so the amount of nickel in a blueberry grown in California may be different from that in a blueberry grown in New York. And the average nickel in an American blueberry may be different from what is in a blueberry in Chile. On average, nickel intake in the United States is 100 mcg/d or less, while the upper limit is estimated at 0.017 mg/kg/d, or 17 mcg/kg/d. The upper limit equates to 1190 mcg/d for a 150 lb adult (about 70kg). Exact levels aside, there are some foods that are consistently high in nickel, regardless of regional differences in soil content.

Tips on What to Eat

- Meat, poultry, and eggs are usually lower in nickel than plant foods are.

- Most fish are good choices, and offer the benefits of healthy fats.

- Dairy products are relatively low in nickel and can be in the diet, including milk, yogurt, cheese, and butter.

- Refined grains, such as white rice, white pasta, and so on, seem to be lower in nickel than whole grains are.

- Vegetables that are lower in nickel include potatoes, cabbage, mushrooms, and cucumber.

- Green leafy vegetables may be high in nickel but are very valuable nutritionally. It may be wise to incorporate small amounts into your diet, and when choosing leafy greens, go for younger leaves because they will have a lower level of nickel than the older leaves.

- Nickel from pipes could possibly transfer to tap water, so letting the water flow for a few seconds before using it may mean lower-nickel water for drinking or cooking.

- You can include citrus fruit and other foods with vitamin C or iron-rich foods, such as tea and coffee, as these foods may decrease how much nickel the body absorbs. But be aware that tea and coffee tend to have moderate levels of nickel, so it's good to include them sparingly, perhaps 1 to 2 cups per day.

- Bananas, apples, and citrus fruit, which are all common in the US diet, can each be eaten a few times a week.

Common High-Nickel Foods

- Baking powder
- Beverages made from high- and medium-nickel foods (e.G., Soy milk, tomato juice)
- Buckwheat
- Canned foods
- Certain vitamin supplements
- Chocolate
- Cocoa
- Dried fruits
- Gelatin
- Legumes (peas, lentils, peanut, soybeans, and chickpeas)
- Millet
- Oat
- Red kidney beans
- Rye
- Soy products
- Strong licorice
- Tea
- Whole grain
- Whole wheat

Common Medium-Nickel Foods

- Beer
- Hazelnuts
- Herring
- Linseeds

- Mackerel
- Marzipan
- Onion
- Raw carrots
- Red wine

- Shellfish
- Sunflower seeds
- Tomatoes
- Tuna
- Walnuts

Tips on What to Avoid

- Avoid all foods from the common high-nickel foods list.

- Read nutrition labels on drinks and vitamin supplements to check for nickel levels.

- Stay away from canned foods.

- Most fish is OK, but some fish can be higher in nickel, including tuna, herring, shellfish, salmon, and mackerel.

- Onion and garlic can be used in moderation, but they do contain some nickel.

- If you use metal utensils, make sure they are not stainless steel or nickel-plated.

- While cooking, avoid cooking with acids (e.g., vinegar, orange juice, lemon juice, or tomatoes) in stainless steel, as it may help nickel transfer to food.

- Please note that the food and beverage industry commonly uses stainless steel in processing that may leech nickel into food; to avoid this nickel, avoid processed foods.

- Anemia should be addressed, both for general health and because it can make the body more receptive to absorbing nickel.

How to Avoid Corn

Corn is fairly simple to avoid as long as you avoid processed and packaged foods. Foods where corn is the main ingredient are obvious: corn on the cob, corn nuts, popcorn, corn chips, vegetable medley including corn. It gets tricky when looking at processed foods with many ingredients. Some of the ingredients are obviously from corn (e.g., cornmeal), but others are less obvious (e.g., modified starch). Corn products contribute thiamine, riboflavin, niacin, iron, and chromium to the diet. Include other whole or enriched grain products that contain these nutrients in your diet. Read all product labels carefully before purchasing and consuming any item. Ingredients in packaged food products may change without warning, so check ingredient statements carefully every time you shop. If you have questions, call the manufacturer.

Foods and Ingredients to Avoid

- Any fats, oils, or salad dressings that contain corn or cornstarch
- Any product prepared with ingredients that contain corn
- Baking powder
- Canned fruit and juice containing corn syrup or high fructose corn syrup
- Caramel
- Caramel corn
- Corn
- Corn alcohol
- Corn flour
- Corn grits
- Corn meal
- Corn or vegetable oil
- Corn sugar
- Corn sweetener
- Corn syrup
- Corn syrup solids
- Corn tortillas
- Cornflakes
- Cornstarch
- Dextrate
- Dextrin
- Dextrose
- Glucose
- Grits
- Hominy
- Maize
- Maltodextrin
- Maltodextrose
- Masa
- Modified gum starch
- Modified starch
- Polenta
- Popcorn
- Sorbitol
- Starch
- Vegetable gum
- Vegetable paste
- Vegetable protein
- Vegetable starch
- Vinegar

Foods that Might Contain Corn (Proceed with Caution)

- Baked goods
- Candies
- Canned and dried soups
- Canned fruits
- Cereals
- Cookies

- Cough drops
- Egg substitutes
- Extracts
- Flavored yogurts
- French bread
- Frozen pancakes
- Fruit drinks and fruit punches
- Ice cream
- Infant formulas
- Jams
- Jellies
- Ketchup
- Luncheon meats
- Margarine
- Packaged potato and pasta products
- Peanut butter

- Powdered coffee creamers
- Processed cheese
- Pudding
- Ramen noodles
- Regular sodas and beverages
- Salad dressing
- Sauces
- Seasonings
- Snack foods
- Spaghetti sauce
- Store-bought baked goods
- Sweetened juices
- Syrups
- Toaster pastries
- Waffles

How to Avoid Eggs

Eggs contribute vitamin B12, riboflavin, pantothenic acid, biotin, and selenium to the diet. When you avoid eggs, you should obtain these nutrients from other foods, such as lean meats, poultry, legumes, and whole or enriched grain products.

Label Smarts

The federal Food Allergen Labeling and Consumer Protection Act (FALCPA) requires that all packaged food products sold in the United States that contain egg as an ingredient must list the word *egg* on the label. The eight major allergens, which must be labeled, are milk, eggs, wheat, peanuts, soy, tree nuts, fish, and shellfish.

Read all product labels carefully before purchasing and consuming any item. Ingredients in packaged food products may change without warning, so check ingredient statements carefully every time you shop. If you have questions, call the manufacturer. Please note that *ovo* means "egg."

Foods and Ingredients to Avoid

- Albumin (albumen)
- Any flavored fruit product with egg ingredients
- Any flavored or seasoned vegetable with egg
- Any product prepared with ingredients that contain egg
- Apoveitellin
- Avidin
- Béarnaise sauce
- Challah
- Egg bread
- Egg matzoh
- Egg noodles
- Egg rolls
- Eggnog
- Eggs in all forms (whole, white, yolk, dried, frozen, powdered, solids, substitutes)
- Flavoprotein
- Globulin
- Hollandaise sauce
- Imitation egg product
- Livetin
- Lysozyme
- Mayonnaise and salad dressings with ingredients that contain egg
- Ovalbumin
- Ovoglobulin
- Ovoglycoprotein
- Ovomucin
- Ovomucoid
- Ovomuxoid
- Prepared meats, poultry, and fish that are flavored or seasoned with egg ingredients
- Simplesse
- Surimi
- Vitellin

Foods that Might Contain Egg (Proceed with Caution)

- Baked goods
- Foam or topping for coffee or cocktails
- Lecithin
- Macaroni
- Marshmallows
- Marzipan

- Nougat
- Pasta

- Pretzels

How to Avoid Cow's Milk

Note: Milk contributes riboflavin, pantothenic acid, vitamin A, vitamin D, phosphorus, and calcium to the diet. When you avoid milk and products that contain milk, you should obtain these nutrients from other foods. Enriched (fortified) soy, potato, or rice milk are good sources of calcium, vitamin A, and vitamin D. Alternative sources of riboflavin, pantothenic acid, and phosphorus include lean meats, legumes, nuts, and whole or enriched grain products.

Label Smarts

The federal Food Allergen Labeling and Consumer Protection Act (FALCPA) requires that all packaged food products sold in the United States that contain milk as an ingredient must list the word *milk* on the label. The eight major allergens, which must be labeled, are milk, eggs, wheat, peanuts, soy, tree nuts, fish, and shellfish.

Read all product labels carefully before purchasing and consuming any item. Ingredients in packaged food products may change without warning, so check ingredient statements carefully every time you shop. If you have questions, call the manufacturer.

If you see *lact-*, *cream*, or *casein*, these are root words for dairy-related ingredients.

Foods and Ingredients to Avoid

- Acidophilus milk
- Butter
- Butter acid
- Butter esters
- Butter oil
- Butterfat
- Buttermilk
- Carob candy
- Casein

- Casein hydrolysate
- Caseinates (in all forms)
- Cheese
- Chocolate milk
- Cottage cheese
- Cream curds
- Creamed candies
- Custard
- Derivative

- Diacetyl
- Dry
- Evaporated
- Ghee
- Goat's milk and milk from other animals
- Half-and-half
- Ice cream
- Including condensed
- Lactalbumin
- Lactalbumin phosphate
- Lactoferrin
- Lactoglobulin
- Lactose
- Lactulose
- Low-fat
- Malted
- Milk (in all forms)
- Milk fat
- Nonfat
- Powder
- Protein

- Protein hydrolysate
- Pudding
- Recaldent
- Rennet casein
- Semisweet chocolate
- Sherbet (most types)
- Simplesse
- Skimmed
- Solids
- Sour cream
- Sour cream solids
- Sour milk solids
- Sweetened condensed milk
- Tagatose
- Whey (in all forms)
- Whey protein hydrolysate
- Whipping cream
- Whole milk protein hydrolysate
- Yogurt
- Yogurt (frozen or regular)

Foods that Might Contain Milk (Proceed with Caution)

- Artificial butter flavor
- Baked goods
- Caramel candies
- Chocolate

- Lactic acid starter culture and other bacterial cultures
- Luncheon meat
- Hot dogs

- Sausages
- Margarine
- Nisin
- Nondairy products
- Nougat
- Bavarian cream flavoring
- Brown sugar flavoring
- Caramel flavoring
- Coconut cream flavoring
- Natural flavoring
- "Cream of anything" soups
- Deli meat (because the slicers are often used to slice both meat and cheese)
- Canned tuna (some contains casein)
- Lots of "nondairy" products list casein in the ingredients
- Some products made with milk substitutes share processing equipment with milk, some meats use casein as a binder (check labels)
- Shellfish is sometimes dipped in milk to reduce fishy odor (ask questions and if you don't get a satisfactory answer, avoid the shellfish)
- Ask how a restaurant prepares its meat and veggies because it may add butter to give them extra flavor
- Some medications have milk protein

Safe Ingredients that Sound as Though They Contain Milk

- Calcium lactate
- Calcium stearoyl lactylate
- Cocoa butter
- Cream of tartar
- Lactic acid
- Oleoresin
- Sodium lactate
- Sodium stearoyl lactylate

How to Avoid Peanuts

Note: Peanuts contribute vitamin E, niacin, magnesium, manganese, and chromium to the diet. When you avoid peanuts and products that contain peanuts, obtain these nutrients from other foods, such as whole or enriched grain products, lean meats and poultry, legumes, and vegetable oils.

Label Smarts

The federal Food Allergen Labeling and Consumer Protection Act (FALCPA) requires that all packaged food products sold in the United States that contain peanut as an ingredient must list the word *peanut* on the label. The eight major allergens, which must be labeled, are milk, eggs, wheat, peanuts, soy, tree nuts, fish, and shellfish.

Read all product labels carefully before purchasing and consuming any item. Ingredients in packaged food products may change without warning, so check ingredient statements carefully every time you shop. If you have questions, call the manufacturer.

Foods and Ingredients to Avoid

- Arachis oil
- Artificial nuts
- Artificial tree nuts
- Beer nuts
- Chopped peanuts
- Cold-pressed peanut oil
- Defatted peanuts
- Egg rolls
- Expelled or expressed peanut oil
- Fresh peanuts
- Goobers
- Granulated peanuts
- Ground nuts
- High-protein food
- Hydrolyzed plant protein
- Hydrolyzed vegetable protein
- Mandelonas
- Marzipan
- Mixed nuts
- Monkey nuts
- Nougat
- Nut meat
- Nut pieces
- Peanut butter
- Peanut flakes
- Peanut flour
- Peanut meal
- Peanut oil
- Peanut protein hydrolysate
- Peanut soup
- Peanuts

Foods that Might Contain Peanuts (Proceed with Caution)

- African, Asian, and Mexican foods
- Baked goods
- Candy
- Cashew butter
- Cheesecake crust
- Chili
- Chili sauce
- Chocolate candy
- Egg rolls
- Foods that contain extruded, cold-pressed, or expelled peanut oil (these may contain peanut protein)

- Frozen desserts
- Glazes and marinades
- Gravy
- Hamster feed
- Hot chocolate
- Hot sauce
- Ice cream
- Ice cream shops
- Livestock feed
- Marzipan
- Molé sauce
- Nougat
- Other nut butters (these can be processed on the same machinery as peanuts, so check the label or even call the manufacturer)

- Pancakes
- Pesto
- Pet food
- Pie crusts
- Pudding
- Salad dressing
- Sauces
- Some vegetarian food products (especially those advertised as meat substitutes)
- Specialty pizzas
- Sunflower seeds (these are often processed on equipment shared with peanuts)

How to Avoid Soy

Note: Soy products contribute thiamine, riboflavin, iron, magnesium, pyridoxine, folacin, calcium, phosphorus, and zinc to the diet. Soy is used in commercial products in small amounts; therefore elimination of soy from the diet should not compromise the nutritional quality of your diet.

Label Smarts

The federal Food Allergen Labeling and Consumer Protection Act (FALCPA) requires that all packaged food products sold in the United States that contain soy as an ingredient must list the word *soy* on the label. The eight major allergens, which must be labeled, are milk, eggs, wheat, peanuts, soy, tree nuts, fish, and shellfish.

Read all product labels carefully before purchasing and consuming any item. Ingredients in packaged food products may change without warning, so check ingredient statements carefully every time you shop. If you have questions, call the manufacturer.

Foods and Ingredients to Avoid

- Chee-fan
- Deep-fried mature soy seed
- Edamame
- Fermented soybean paste
- Fermented soybeans
- Hamanatto
- Ketjap
- Metiauza
- Miso
- Natto
- Soy (soy albumin)
- Soy cheese
- Soy fiber
- Soy flour
- Soy grits
- Soy ice cream
- Soy milk
- Soy nuts
- Soy protein (concentrate, hydrolyzed, isolate)
- Soy protein shakes
- Soy sauce (shoyu)
- Soy sprouts
- Soy yogurt
- Soya
- Soybean (curd, granules)
- Soybean sprouts
- Sufu
- Tamari
- Tao-cho
- Tao-si
- Taotjo
- Tempeh
- Textured soy protein
- Textured vegetable protein (TVP)
- Tofu
- Whey-soy drink

Foods that Might Contain Soy

- Asian cuisine
- Baked goods
- Breakfast cereal
- Canned tuna and meat
- Cookies
- Crackers
- High-protein energy bars and snacks
- Hydrolyzed plant protein
- Hydrolyzed vegetable protein
- Infant formulas
- Low-fat peanut butter
- Natural flavoring

- Packaged meals
- Sauces
- Soups

- Vegetable broth
- Vegetable gum
- Vegetable starch

How to Avoid Wheat

Note: Wheat provides a good source of thiamine, riboflavin, niacin, iron, selenium, and chromium. Whole or enriched alternative grains, such as oats, rice, rye, barley, corn, buckwheat, amaranth, and quinoa, contain these nutrients.

Label Smarts

The federal Food Allergen Labeling and Consumer Protection Act (FALCPA) requires that all packaged food products sold in the United States that contain wheat as an ingredient must list the word *wheat* on the label. The eight major allergens, which must be labeled, are milk, eggs, wheat, peanuts, soy, tree nuts, fish, and shellfish.

Read all product labels carefully before purchasing and consuming any item. Ingredients in packaged food products may change without warning, so check ingredient statements carefully every time you shop. If you have questions, call the manufacturer.

Buckwheat is not wheat. Instead, it is a gluten-free whole grain that makes delicious crepes, pancakes, and cold noodle salads.

Foods and Ingredients to Avoid

- Acker meal
- Atta
- Bal haar
- Bran
- Bread
- Bread crumbs
- Bread flour
- Bulgur
- Cake flour
- Cereal extract

- Club wheat
- Couscous
- Cracker meal
- Doughnuts
- Durum
- Einkorn
- Emmer
- Farina
- Flour (all-purpose, bread, cake, durum, enriched, graham, high-gluten, high-

protein, instant, pastry, self-rising, soft wheat, steel ground, stone ground, whole wheat)

- Hydrolyzed wheat protein
- Kamut (a brand of khorasan wheat)
- Matzo
- Matzo meal (also spelled matzoh)
- Multigrain breads
- Multigrain flours
- Pasta
- Pastries
- Pies
- Puffed wheat
- Red wheat flakes
- Rolled wheat
- Seitan
- Semolina
- Shredded wheat
- Soft wheat flour
- Spelt
- Sprouted wheat
- Superamine
- Tortillas
- Triticale
- Vital gluten
- Vital wheat gluten
- Vitalia macaroni

- Wheat (bran, durum, germ, gluten, grass, malt, sprouts, starch)
- Wheat bran
- Wheat bran hydrolysate
- Wheat bread
- Wheat bread crumbs
- Wheat flakes
- Wheat germ
- Wheat germ oil
- Wheat gluten
- Wheat grass
- Wheat malt
- Wheat meal
- Wheat pasta
- Wheat protein beverage
- Wheat protein isolate
- Wheat protein powder
- Wheat starch
- Wheat tempeh
- White flour
- Whole wheat berries
- Whole wheat flour
- Winter wheat flour

Foods that Might Contain Wheat (Proceed with Caution)

- Gelatinized starch
- Glucose syrup
- Gluten
- High-gluten flour
- High-protein flour

- Hydrolyzed vegetable protein
- Modified food starch
- Modified starch
- Soy sauce

- Starch
- Surimi
- Vegetable gum
- Vegetable starch

How to Avoid Tree Nuts

Note: Tree nuts are a good source of vitamin E, magnesium, copper, manganese, and omega-3 fatty acids. A varied diet, which includes lean meats and poultry, seafood, fruits, vegetables, whole or enriched grain products, legumes, and vegetable oil, can provide these nutrients. A tree nut–free diet should not result in any nutrient deficiencies.

Label Smarts

The federal Food Allergen Labeling and Consumer Protection Act (FALCPA) requires that all packaged food products sold in the United States that contain tree nuts as an ingredient must list the specific tree nut used on the label. The eight major allergens, which must be labeled, are milk, eggs, wheat, peanuts, soy, tree nuts, fish, and shellfish.

Read all product labels carefully before purchasing and consuming any item. Ingredients in packaged food products may change without warning, so check ingredient statements carefully every time you shop. If you have questions, call the manufacturer.

There is no evidence that products made from coconuts and shea nuts, which are on the FDA "tree nut" list and are allergenic compared to other tree nuts; products include coconut oil, coconut butter, shea nut oil, or shea nut butter. Nutmeg is not a nut.

Foods and Ingredients to Avoid

- Almond
- Artificial nuts
- Beechnut
- Brazil nut
- Butternut

- Cashew
- Chestnut
- Chinquapin nut
- Coconut
- Gianduja (a chocolate-nut mixture)

- Ginkgo nut

- Hazelnut (filbert) hickory nut

- Lichee (alternative spellings are litchi, lychee, and lichi) nut

- Macadamia nut

- Marzipan (almond paste)

- Nangai nut

- Natural nut extract (e.g., almond, walnut)

- Nut butters (e.g., cashew butter)

- Nut meal

- Nut meat

- Nut paste (e.g., almond paste)

- Nut pieces

- Pecan

- Pesto

- Pili nut

- Pine nut (also referred to as Indian, pignoli, pignolia, pignon, piñon, and pinyon nut)

- Pistachio

- Praline

- Shea nut

- Walnut

Foods that Might Contain Tree Nuts (Proceed with Caution)

- Asian foods

- Baked goods

- Baking mixes

- Black walnut hull extract (flavoring)

- Breading

- Desserts

- Ice cream toppings

- Natural nut extract

- Nut distillates (alcoholic extracts)

- Nut oils (e.g., walnut oil, almond oil)

- Salads

- Sauces

- Walnut hull extract (flavoring)

How to Avoid Fish

Note: Fish contributes niacin, vitamin B6, vitamin B12, vitamin E, phosphorus, omega-3 fatty acids, and selenium to the diet. When you avoid eating fish and products that contain fish or fish proteins, you should obtain these nutrients from other foods, such as lean meats and poultry, whole grains, flax seed, legumes, walnuts, Brazil nuts, and vegetable oils.

Label Smarts

The federal Food Allergen Labeling and Consumer Protection Act (FALCPA) requires that all packaged food products sold in the United States that contain fish as an ingredient must list the specific fish used on the label. The eight major allergens, which must be labeled, are milk, eggs, wheat, peanuts, soy, tree nuts, fish, and shellfish.

Read all product labels carefully before purchasing and consuming any item. Ingredients in packaged food products may change without warning, so check ingredient statements carefully every time you shop. If you have questions, call the manufacturer.

Fish protein can become airborne in the steam released during cooking and may be a risk. If you are sensitive to it, stay away from cooking areas.

Foods and Ingredients to Avoid

- All fish
- Anchovies
- Bass
- Catfish
- Cod
- Fish stock
- Flounder
- Grouper
- Haddock
- Hake
- Halibut
- Herring
- Mahimahi
- Perch
- Pike
- Pollock
- Salmon
- Scrod
- Snapper
- Sole
- Swordfish
- Tilapia
- Trout
- Tuna

Foods that Might Contain Fish

- Barbecue sauce
- Beer
- Bouillabaisse
- Caesar salad and dressing
- Caponata
- Imitation or artificial fish or shellfish (surimi)
- Meat loaf
- Wine
- Worcestershire sauce

How to Avoid Shellfish

Note: Shellfish contributes zinc, magnesium, copper, and selenium to the diet. When you avoid shellfish, you should obtain these nutrients from other foods, such as lean meats, eggs, whole or enriched grain products, seeds, fruits, and vegetables.

Label Smarts

The federal Food Allergen Labeling and Consumer Protection Act (FALCPA) requires that all packaged food products sold in the United States that contain shellfish as an ingredient must list the specific shellfish used on the label. The eight major allergens, which must be labeled, are milk, eggs, wheat, peanuts, soy, tree nuts, fish, and shellfish.

Read all product labels carefully before purchasing and consuming any item. Ingredients in packaged food products may change without warning, so check ingredient statements carefully every time you shop. If you have questions, call the manufacturer.

Any food served in a seafood restaurant may contain shellfish protein due to cross-contact.

Foods and Ingredients to Avoid

- Barnacle
- Crab
- Crawfish (crawdad, crayfish, ecrevisse)
- Krill
- Lobster (langouste, langoustine, moreton bay bugs, scampi, tomalley)
- Prawns
- Shrimp (crevette, scampi)

Foods that Might Contain Shellfish

- Bouillabaisse
- Cuttlefish ink
- Fish stock
- Glucosamine
- Seafood flavoring (e.g., crab or clam extract)
- Surimi

CHAPTER 17

Maintenance Diet Tools

Daily Food Plans

The USDA has different levels of calories, and your daily intake for each food group is based on age, gender, height, weight, and physical activity level. The standard 2000-calorie diet is a benchmark used by the FDA for food labels. All food plans below are for adults 18 years and older.

Daily Food Plan Guidelines for Your Maintenance Diet

	Protein	Calcium-Rich Foods	Grains and Starches	Vegetables	Fruits	Oils
Lower: 1,600 calories	5 oz	3 cups	5 oz	2 cups	1.5 cups	5 tsp
Lower: 1,800 calories	5 oz	3 cups	6 oz	2.5 cups	1.5 cups	5 tsp
Standard: 2,000 calories	5.5 oz	3 cups	6 oz	2.5 cups	2 cups	6 tsp
Higher: 2,200 calories	6 oz	3 cups	7 oz	3 cups	2 cups	6 tsp
Higher: 2,400 calories	6.5 oz	3 cups	8 oz	3 cups	2 cups	7 tsp
Higher: 2,600 calories	6.5 oz	3 cups	9 oz	3.5 cups	2 cups	8 tsp
Higher: 2,800 calories	7 oz	3 cups	10 oz	3.5 cups	2.5 cups	8 tsp
Higher: 3,000 calories	7 oz	3 cups	10 oz	4 cups	2.5 cups	10 tsp
Higher: 3,200 calories	7 oz	3 cups	10 oz	4 cups	2.5 cups	11 tsp

Foods for Your Maintenance Plan

Protein

Meat
Beef, bison, buffalo, lamb, pork, rabbit, veal, venison

Poultry
Chicken, duck, goose, quail, turkey

Eggs
Chicken, duck, quail, turkey, goose

Fish
Anchovy, catfish, cod, flounder, haddock, halibut, herring, mackerel, pollock, salmon, sardines, sea bass, snapper, sole, swordfish, tilapia, trout, tuna

Shellfish
Clams, crabs, crayfish, lobsters, mussels, oysters, prawns, scallops, shrimp

Milk
Cow, goat, sheep, soy

Dairy
Cheese, yogurt

Nuts and Seeds
Almonds, cashews, hazelnuts, pecans, pistachios, pumpkin seeds, sunflower seeds, walnuts

Beans
Adzuki beans, black-eyed peas, black beans, kidney beans, lentils, lima beans, navy beans, peanuts, pinto beans, soybeans, split peas, tempeh, tofu, white beans, yellow beans

Grains and Starches

Grains (often come in whole forms as well as breads, pastas, crackers, tortillas, and cereal)
Amaranth, barley, brown rice, buckwheat groats, bulgur, corn pasta, couscous, Kamut, millet, oat bran, oats, oatmeal, popcorn, quinoa, rye, spinach spaghetti, spelt, teff, triticale, whole grain bread, whole wheat noodles, wild rice

Starchy Vegetables (Roots, Tubers, Plantains)

Beans (broad beans, butter beans, dried peas, garbanzo beans, lentils, lima beans, soybeans), beets, carrots, cassava, corn, green peas, parsnips, plantains, potatoes, pumpkin, parsnips, sweet potatoes, tapioca, taro, winter squash (e.g., acorn, butternut, kabocha), yams

Vegetables

Greens

Artichokes, arugula, asparagus, avocados, basil, beet greens, broccoli, broccoli rabe, broccoflower, Brussels sprouts, bok choy, cabbage, celery, chayote squash, Chinese cabbage, cilantro, collard greens, cucumbers, edamame, endive, escarole, fennel, green beans, green olives, green peppers, green peas, jalapeño, kale, lettuce, mâche lettuce, mustard greens, okra, other leafy greens or herbs, parsley, radish greens, spinach, sprouts, Swiss chard, turnip greens, tomatillos, watercress, zucchini

Beans and peas

French beans (haricots vert), green beans, green peas, snap peas, snow peas, string beans, sugar peas

Blues, purples, and reds

Beets, Belgian endive, black olives, black salsify, eggplant, Okinawan sweet potato, purple carrots, radicchio, red cabbage, red pepper, red tomato, red onion, rhubarb, red beans, red potatoes, purple peppers, purple asparagus, shallots

Yellows and oranges

Acorn squash, butternut squash, carrots, corn, pumpkins, rutabagas, spaghetti squash, sweet potatoes, yellow beets, yellow peppers, yellow squash, yellow tomatoes, yellow potatoes

White, tan, and brown

Cauliflower, garlic, onions, radishes, green onion, chives, ginger, mushrooms, jicama, potatoes, white beans, turnips, parsnips, white asparagus, kohlrabi, shallots, white corn, water chestnuts

Fruit

Citrus: Vitamin C

Grapefruit (pink, white), kumquat, lemon (Meyer), lime (key, Kaffir), Mandarin orange, orange (Mineola, Seville, juice, navel, blood), pummelo, tangelo, tangerine (satsuma)

Vine fruits

Cantaloupe, grapes or raisins (green, purple, black, Concord), honeydew, melon (Canary, Crenshaw), watermelon (red, yellow)

Berries: anthocyanins, vitamin C

Blackberries, black currants, blueberries, boysenberries, Cape gooseberries, cranberries, elderberries, gooseberries, raspberries, strawberries

Tree fruit

Apples (honey crisp, Fuji, Pink Lady, red, green, Crispin, Braeburn, Golden Delicious), figs, pears (green, Bosc, Starkrimson), pomegranate

Tropical or Asian fruit

Avocados, bananas, dates, dragon fruit, guavas, lichee fruit, mangoes, papayas, pineapple, starfruit, Asian pears, fuyu persimmons, passion fruit, açai, kiwifruit (golden, green)

Stone fruit

Apricots, apriums, pluots, cherries (red, bing), nectarines (white, yellow), peaches (white, yellow), plums, prunes

Healthy Oils

Healthy oils from food

Almonds, avocados, fatty fish (salmon, tuna, sardines, trout, herring, mackerel), flax, olives, pistachios, walnuts

Healthy oils

Canola oil, olive oil, safflower oil, sunflower oil, vegetable oil

Appendix

Resources

Find a Registered Dietitian

The Academy of Nutrition and Dietetics (formerly the American Dietetic Association) was founded in 1917 and is the world's largest organization of food and nutrition professionals. The Academy is committed to improving the nation's health and advancing the profession of dietetics through research, education, and advocacy. They house a handy searchable database of registered dietitians (RDs), which you can search by zip code or even by expertise. Visit them at www.eatright.org/programs/rdfinder. For example, you can find RDs with expertise in digestive disorders, food allergies and intolerances, or gluten intolerance. You can also filter results by language, including Chinese, French, Hindi, Korean, Spanish, Tagalog, and more.

Find a Support Group for Food Allergies

The Asthma and Allergy Foundation of America (AAFA) was founded in 1953 and is the leading patient organization for people with asthma and allergies. AAFA is the oldest asthma and allergy patient group in the world. They have educational support groups across the country to help you gather relevant information about asthma and allergies and to offer emotional support. The groups, although not identical, all offer guest speakers, a medical adviser, and a face-to-face supportive environment to share information and solutions for managing asthma and allergies. AAFA offers four types of groups, based on audience: one for parents, one for preteens, one for teens, and one for adults, by specific food allergies. You can find a support group by state at www.aafa.org/esg_search.cfm. The food allergy groups are formed in partnership with Food Allergy Research and Education (FARE).

The Food Allergy Research and Education (FARE) organization works on behalf of the 15 million Americans with food allergies, including those at risk for life-threatening anaphylaxis. According to FARE, food allergies affect 1 in 13 children in the United States. FARE was formed in 2012 as a merger between the Food Allergy and Anaphylaxis Network (FAAN) and the Food Allergy Initiative (FAI). They are an excellent source of information on many aspects of food allergies, including less common allergies. They can also help you find a support group near you by country and state; visit them at www. foodallergy.org/support-groups.

Find an Allergist

The American Academy of Allergy, Asthma, and Immunology (AAAAI) is a professional organization with more than 6,700 members in the United States, Canada, and 72 other countries. This membership includes allergists, immunologists, other medical specialists, and allied health and related health care professionals—all with a special interest in the research and treatment of allergic and immunologic diseases. They offer a way to find an allergist through an interactive map, which you can filter by zip code, name search, or geographic search. Visit the American Academy of Allergy, Asthma and Immunology at www.aaaai.org.

The American College of Allergy, Asthma, and Immunology (ACAAI) is also a professional organization. Composed of allergists, immunologists, and allied health professionals, they were established in 1942 and count more than 5,700 members. They promote excellence in the practice of the subspecialty of allergy and immunology and offer five-year board certification programs for physicians. You can find an allergist by city or zip code, and you can also filter your results by distance radius, specialty area, or name; the results will list languages spoken by the allergist and whether he or she accepts pediatric or adult patients or both. Visit them at www.acaai.org/allergist/Pages/locate_an_allergist.aspx.

The Jaffe Food Allergy Institute is a well-respected food allergy clinical and research center housed in the Icahn School of Medicine at Mount Sinai in New York City. The mission of the institute is to expand and improve basic science and clinical research, comprehensive patient care, and educational efforts in the field of food allergy. Institute members conduct basic science and clinical research activities related to food allergic disorders; provide comprehensive clinical care for food allergy patients; conduct educational programs related to food allergic disorders for physicians and other health care professionals, patients, families, and the general public; and develop or collaborate on additional programs, including publications, symposia, patient education programs, and curriculum development and testing for health care professionals. The institute's phone number is 212-241-5749. You can also learn more about the institute here: icahn.mssm.edu/research/programs/jaffe-food-allergy-institute.

Find a Certified LEAP Therapist (CLT)

The certified LEAP therapist (CLT) is a specialist in non-IgE food sensitivity treatment and therapy. A CLT uses the LEAP elimination diet, based on the mediator release test (MRT) test results and client history, to develop the most effective anti-inflammatory elimination diet. If it's not an elimination diet, it's not a LEAP diet.

Certification is obtained via a 30-hour-plus LEAP therapist training, which is a combination of self-study, experience, and working one-on-one with an experienced CLT LEAP mentor.

Be Informed

Sign up for food recall alerts from the FDA. Many of the recalls are related to undeclared allergens making their way into foods. For example, flavored potato chips may contain milk but accidentally make it to the grocery shelf without milk being listed in the ingredients. When this is discovered, the manufacturer will send out a recall notice. Sometimes this makes the news, but not always, as there are several recalls a day. To get all the notices, sign up for email alerts by visiting www.fda.gov/safety/recalls and clicking on the link that says, "Sign up to receive Recalls, Market Withdrawals, & Safety Alerts." This page will also list recently posted recalls.

As part of the USDA's National Agricultural Library, Nutrition.gov is a free resource, providing easy access to vetted food and nutrition information from across the federal government to consumers. Staff there serve as a gateway and a clearinghouse for reliable information on nutrition and healthy eating. Of particular interest, they have information categorized under "food allergies and intolerances" at www.nutrition.gov/nutrition-and-health-issues/food-allergies-and-intolerances, as well as under "digestive disorders" at www.nutrition.gov/nutrition-and-health-issues/digestive-disorders. In addition, they link out to more in-depth information from the USDA's Food and Nutrition Information Center (FNIC), which is heavily staffed by RDs. Staff at the center provide information on allergies and food sensitivities at fnic.nal.usda.gov/diet-and-disease/allergies-and-food-sensitivities, and also provide more information about digestive diseases and disorders at fnic.nal.usda.gov/diet-and-disease/digestive-diseases-and-disorders.

An informative guide to managing food allergies is available for free from the National Institute of Allergy and Infectious Diseases (NIAID), part of the National Institutes of Health. Staff there undertook a two-year effort, working with thirty-four professional organizations, federal agencies, and patient advocacy groups to develop guidelines for diagnosing and managing food allergies in the United States. The guide was published in December 2010. The primary audience for the guidelines is health care professionals, but they also created a consumer guide for patients, families, and caregivers that is available online at: www.niaid.nih.gov/topics/foodAllergy/clinical/Documents/FAguidelinesPatient.pdf. The same NIAID created a short, informative video to illustrate how food allergies work, and it is available on the NIAID YouTube channel here: youtube.com/user/niaid.

Glossary

Allergy, immunoglobulin E (IgE) mediated, is an allergy whose symptoms are the result of interaction between an allergen and a type of antibody known as IgE, which is thought to play a major role in allergic reactions, e.g., milk allergy.

Allergy, non-IgE-mediated, is an allergy whose symptoms are the result of interaction of the allergen with the immune system, but the interaction does not involve an IgE antibody, e.g., celiac disease.

An **allergen** is a protein substance that can cause an allergic reaction. In some people, the immune system thinks allergens are foreign or dangerous. This is what leads to allergy symptoms.

Allergic proctocolitis (AP), is a disorder that occurs in infants who seem healthy but have visible specks or streaks of blood mixed with mucus in their stool. Because there are no laboratory tests to diagnose food-induced AP, a health care professional must rely on a medical history showing that certain foods cause symptoms to occur. Many infants have AP while being breast-fed, probably because the mother's milk contains food proteins from her diet that cause an allergic reaction in the infant.

Anaphylaxis is a serious allergic reaction that involves more than one body system (for example, skin and respiratory tract or gastrointestinal tract or all three body systems), begins very rapidly, and may cause death.

Angioedema is swelling due to fluid collecting under the skin, in the abdominal organs, or in the upper airway (nose, back of the throat, or voice box). It often occurs with hives and, if caused by food, is typically IgE-mediated. When the upper airway is involved, swelling in the voice box is an emergency, requiring immediate medical attention. Acute angioedema is a common feature of anaphylaxis.

Contact urticaria (hives) occur when the skin comes in contact with an allergen. The hives can be local or widespread. They are caused by antibodies interacting with allergen proteins or from the direct release of histamine, a molecule involved in allergy.

Cross-reactive foods are foods that are seen as similar to allergenic foods by the immune system. An antibody that reacts with the allergenic food also reacts with the cross-reactive food. For example, a person who is allergic to shrimp may also be allergic to lobster, because shrimp and lobster are closely related foods. In this case, lobster would be a cross-reactive food.

Dermatitis, allergic contact (ACD), is a form of eczema caused by an allergic reaction to food additives or molecules that occur naturally in foods, such as mangoes. The allergic reaction involves immune cells but not IgE-type antibodies. Symptoms include itching, redness, swelling, and small raised areas on the skin that may or may not contain fluid.

Dermatitis, contact, is an inflammation of the skin in which the skin becomes red, sore, or inflamed after direct contact with a substance. There are two kinds of contact dermatitis: irritant and allergic.

Dermatitis, systemic contact, is a rare disorder with symptoms that include eczema, fever, headache, and stuffy nose. To develop systemic contact dermatitis, a person first develops specific IgE antibodies to the allergen through contact with the skin. If the person subsequently swallows the allergen or is exposed to it though a skin cut or puncture, symptoms develop.

Eczema (atopic dermatitis or atopic eczema) is a disease of the skin. Symptoms include scaly, itchy rashes and blistering, weeping, or peeling of the skin. The causes of the disease are unclear. There may be a problem in the skin's ability to maintain an effective barrier against environmental factors, such as irritants, microbes, and allergens. A person who has a biological parent or sibling with a history of allergy or eczema is at risk for developing food allergy.

Elimination Diet, Catchall is a diet that eliminates most foods and instead focuses on a relatively small set of foods that are allowed. The ultimate goal of this diet is also to identify food sensitivities. The Catchall Elimination Diet may be helpful if Targeted Elimination Diets have not worked or if it's unclear what the possible offending food is.

Elimination Diet, Targeted is a diet that targets a set of foods to eliminate from the diet in order to identify food sensitivities. A Targeted Elimination Diet might eliminate only one food or it could be many foods.

Enterocolitis is an inflammation of the colon and small intestine.

Enteropathy is a disease of the intestine.

Eosinophilic esophagitis (EoE) is a disorder associated with food allergy, but how it is related is unclear. It occurs when types of immune cells called eosinophils collect in the esophagus. Both IgE- and non-IgE-mediated mechanisms appear to be involved in EoE.

Epinephrine (adrenaline) is a hormone that increases heart rate, tightens the blood vessels, and opens the airways. Epinephrine is the best treatment for anaphylaxis.

Exercise-induced anaphylaxis is a type of severe, whole-body allergic reaction that occurs during physical activity. Food is the trigger in about one-third of patients who have experienced exercise-induced anaphylaxis. This reaction is likely to recur in patients.

FODMAPs-based elimination diet is a diet that eliminates FODMAPs, which stands for Fermentable Oligo-, Di-, and Monosaccharides, And Polyols, which are poorly digested carbohydrates that sometimes cause abdominal pain, bloating, and diarrhea in prone people.

A **food allergy** is caused by the immune system reacting to a food in a way that it shouldn't. Symptoms come from a specific immune response to a given food, called an allergen.

A **food intolerance**, or a food sensitivity, occurs when a person has difficulty digesting a particular food that does not involve the immune system. This can lead to symptoms, such as intestinal gas, abdominal pain, or diarrhea.

Food sensitivity is a generic term that can be used to describe a variety of negative reactions to a food; this term could be used to describe either an allergy or an intolerance.

Food protein-induced enterocolitis syndrome (FPIES) is a non-IgE-mediated disorder that usually occurs in young infants. Symptoms include chronic vomiting, diarrhea, and failure to gain weight or height. When the allergenic food is removed from the infant's diet, symptoms disappear. Milk and soy protein are the most common causes, but some studies report reactions to rice, oats, or other cereal grains. A similar condition also has been reported in adults, most often related to eating crustacean shellfish.

GAPS™ diet stands for Gut and Psychology Syndrome™diet, developed by Dr. Campbell-Mcbride, and is based on the specific carbohydrate diet, which is a diet that removes most carbohydrates from the diet with the rationale that the eliminated carbohydrates are difficult to digest and cause inflammation in the gut.

Prebiotics are natural, nondigestible food ingredients that promote the growth of helpful bacteria in the gut. A prebiotic is a food ingredient that selectively stimulates the growth of microbial species in the gut microbiota that confer health benefits on the host.

Probiotics are live microorganisms (in most cases, bacteria) that are similar to beneficial microorganisms found in the human gut. They are also called friendly bacteria or good bacteria. Probiotics are available to consumers mainly in the form of dietary supplements and foods.

Synbiotic products contain both probiotics and prebiotics.

Meal Planner for the Targeted Elimination Diet

	Breakfast	Lunch/Dinner	Lunch/Dinner	Snacks
Monday				
Tuesday				
Wednesday				
Thursday				
Friday				
Saturday				
Sunday				

Food and Symptom Tracker

Meal	Food/Drink (How Much)	Ingredients	Symptoms
Breakfast Time:			Symptoms: Start time: End time: Rating:
AM Snack Time:			Symptoms: Start time: End time: Rating:
Lunch Time:			Symptoms: Start time: End time: Rating:
PM Snack Time:			Symptoms: Start time: End time: Rating:
Dinner Time:			Symptoms: Start time: End time: Rating:
PM Snack Time:			Symptoms: Start time: End time: Rating:

Index

About the Author

Maggie Moon, MS, RD, is a registered dietitian, nutrition educator, and writer with experience in health communications and supermarket dietetics. An authority on nutrition, health, and wellness, she has been an adjunct lecturer in the Department of Health and Nutrition Sciences at Brooklyn College in New York City, and has served on executive committees for regional and national dietetics associations. She is a graduate of the University of California at Berkeley and received her master of science degree in nutrition education from Columbia University, with clinical training completed at New York–Presbyterian Hospital of Columbia and Cornell.

CPSIA information can be obtained
at www.ICGtesting.com
Printed in the USA
JSHW031252210421
13718JS00001B/1

9 781612 433004